The Biopsychosocial
Formulation Manual

The Biopsychosocial Formulation Manual

A Guide for Mental Health Professionals

William H. Campbell
Robert M. Rohrbaugh

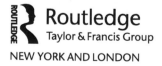

Routledge
Taylor & Francis Group

NEW YORK AND LONDON

Published in 2006 by
Routledge
Taylor & Francis Group
711 Third Avenue,
New York, NY 10017

Published in Great Britain by
Routledge
Taylor & Francis Group
2 Park Square, Milton Park,
Abingdon, Oxfordshire
OX14 4RN

Routledge is an imprint of the Taylor and Francis Group, an informa business

International Standard Book Number-13: 978-1-138-17092-6 (hardcover)
International Standard Book Number-13: 978-0-415-95142-5 (Softcover)
Library of Congress Card Number 2005020806

Library of Congress Cataloging-in-Publication Data

Campbell, William H., 1955-
    The biopsychosocial formulation manual : a guide for mental health professionals / William H. Campbell, Robert M. Rohrbaugh.
        p. ; cm.
    Includes bibliographical references and index.
    ISBN 0-415-95142-9 (pbk.)
    1. Clinical health psychology.   I. Rohrbaugh, Robert M. II. Title.   [DNLM: 1. Mental Disorders--diagnosis. 2. Interview, Psychological. 3. Mental Disorders--therapy. 4. Models, Biological. 5. Models, Psychological. 6. Social Environment.   WM 140 C192b 2006]

R726.7.C36 2006
616.89--dc22   2005020806

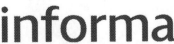

Taylor & Francis Group
is the Academic Division of Informa plc.

Visit the Taylor & Francis Web site at
http://www.taylorandfrancis.com

and the Routledge Web site at
http://www.routledge-ny.com

Contents

Introduction

In 1977, Dr. George Engel's seminal article on the biopsycho-social model of disease, "The Need for a New Medical Model: A Challenge for Biomedicine," was published in *Science*. Over 20 years later, the article is still required reading in many training programs in psychiatry, nursing, psychology, and social work, because the biopsychosocial model advances a comprehensive understanding of disease and treatment. The model is derived from general systems theory, which proposes that each system affects and is affected by the other systems. In the biopsychosocial model, the biological system empha-sizes the anatomical, structural, and molecular substrates of disease and their effects on the patient's* biological function-

---

* The term "patient" will be used throughout this manual in place of "client" to empha-size the importance and uniqueness of the clinician–patient relationship. We view health care as a profession, not a trade, and therefore eschew any reference to the term "client" in this text. It is our belief that patients should be treated with the utmost respect for their dignity and autonomy. In keeping with this view, we fully endorse the principle of informed consent. Disclosing relevant information and educating our patients using terms they can understand is key to establishing a truly collaborative relationship.

ing; the psychological system addresses the contributions of developmental factors, motivation, and personality on the patient's experiences of and reactions to illness; and the social system examines the cultural, environmental, and familial influences on the expression of, as well as the patient's experiences of, illness.

Faculty members in departments of psychiatry, nursing, psychology, and social work typically invest considerable time and effort in teaching their trainees how to interview patients. Although interviewing is a process that is continually refined throughout one's career, trainees soon find themselves capable of eliciting a reasonably comprehensive database from their patient interviews. However, having obtained the requisite data, they find organizing the information in a meaningful way to be an altogether different challenge. The predominant mode of instruction in many contemporary training programs does a disservice to the biopsychosocial model. Depending on the orientation of the discipline (i.e., psychiatry, nursing, psychology, or social work), the formulation emphasized to respective trainees focuses predominantly, and in some instances exclusively, on one or at most two of the three components. This approach limits the development of a truly comprehensive formulation and adversely impacts patient care.

Our goal in developing this manual was to provide trainees (as well as more experienced clinicians) in the mental health professions with a practical approach to organizing the wealth of data obtained from a patient into a meaningful formulation. Using the suggested format, trainees can learn to construct a formulation that ensures appropriate emphasis of all three components (i.e., biological, psychological, and social). To accomplish our goal, we first provide an overview of Engel's biopsychosocial model (Engel, 1980) and then analyze each of the three components. In each of the component sections, we review the information we believe should be included in a comprehensive formulation (the "database"). In the psychological section, we also briefly review the aspects of cognitive, behavioral, and psychodynamic theory that we feel are pertinent to this model of formulation. Experts may question why certain data were included or excluded or why one part of a theory was addressed and another was not. It was necessary to make these judgments while developing a model and a manual that would be practical for trainees beginning their careers in mental health care. We encourage those using this manual to expand those components in a way that is most relevant to their practice.

A database sheet is provided to assist the clinician in recording the interview data into each of three databases.

Each database is then analyzed and further organized to assist the clinician in providing a comprehensive formulation, including a summary of the data, additional information needed (i.e., further history, diagnostic studies), and recommended therapeutic interventions. We believe that this will greatly assist clinicians in their written intake evaluations as well as in their oral presentations.

This model has been used for training psychiatry residents for over 10 years and has been taught in a course format at the American Psychiatric Association's (APA) annual meetings. Evaluations and feedback from our residents and the APA courses exceeded our expectations and served as the initial impetus for us to write this *Biopsychosocial Formulation Manual*. We will continue to refine the manual over time but realize that, as with all works, its most valuable future revisions will result from the feedback obtained from those using it. We hope that you find this manual and the accompanying CD to be valuable learning tools. Enjoy the process — we look forward to hearing from you.

William H. Campbell
Department of Psychiatry
University Hospitals of Cleveland
11100 Euclid Avenue
Cleveland, OH 44106
William.Campbell@uhhs.com

Robert M. Rohrbaugh
Department of Psychiatry
Yale University School of Medicine
300 George Street
Suite 901
New Haven, CT 06511
Robert.Rohrbaugh@yale.edu

I

An Overview of the Biopsychosocial Formulation Model

Many of us have had the experience of observing senior clinicians develop an awe-inspiring formulation after hearing a case presentation. The formulation organizes the patient's presenting symptoms, facilitates an understanding of the genesis of the difficulties, and enables the development of a comprehensive care management plan for ongoing work with the patient. Many beginning clinicians wonder, "How did they do that?" Although trainees read the standard textbooks and study the *Diagnostic and Statistical Manual of Mental Disorders* (*DSM*), the process of organizing the patient data in a meaningful way and marrying it with the theory in an effort to explicate the patient's difficulties eludes them. There is so much information from the patient and the literature that it is difficult to imagine generating a comprehensive biopsychosocial formulation. This manual was written with that purpose in mind.

The *Biopsychosocial Formulation Manual* will assist clinicians by providing them with a structured paradigm to follow both in the initial collection and organization of patient data and in the process of crafting the data into a biopsychosocial formulation. The manual is not meant to take the place of a comprehensive textbook or the *DSM*. Students will need to know the symptoms and diagnostic criteria for mental disorders and have an understanding of the biological, psychological, and social theories that pertain to mental illness. We hope that by identifying the range of pertinent data, organizing the data, and providing a framework for analysis of that data, our readers will become more proficient and confident in their ability to develop biopsychosocial formulations.

The most efficient way to teach a new model is first to provide the student with a bird's-eye view, so they can gain the proper perspective, and then to break the model down into its component parts for further study. Our model is comprised of seven sections: Biological Formulation, Psychological Formulation, Social Formulation, Differential Diagnosis, Risk Assessment, Biopsychosocial Treatment Plan, and Prognosis. The basic outline of the Biopsychosocial Formulation Model appears in Figure 1.1. It is our hope that as you use this manual, you will memorize the model so that it will become an internal mental template that you keep in mind as you evaluate all your patients.

A careful review of all seven sections will provide you with an overview of the data required to construct a comprehensive biopsychosocial formulation. A useful exercise at this point is to ask yourself how much of this data you routinely utilize in your current patient formulations. If you find there are a lot of gaps in your typical formulation, do not be discouraged, you are not alone. The purpose of this manual is to help you develop the skills to collect data and more fully utilize the data you collect.

The process of formulation begins by collecting and organizing patient data from the patient interview and chart review. The Biopsychosocial Formulation Database Record

I.   Biological Formulation

Creation of a Biological/Descriptive Database

A.   What symptoms are elicited?

Mood   Anxiety   Psychotic   Somatic

Cognitive   Substance   Personality   Other

B.   What biological predispositions are present?

1.   Genetics
2.   Physical conditions
3.   Medications/Substances

C.   Do the demographics of the patient match the known
          epidemiology of the disorder(s) under consideration?

II.   Psychological Formulation

A.   General Psychological Formulation

1.   Identifying Psychological Vulnerabilities

a.   Disruptions in psychological development
b.   Revelatory statements and behavior
c.   Recurrent difficulties in relationships (past, current, and with
          therapist)

2.   Identifying Psychosocial Stressors

FIGURE 1.1
The Biopsychosocial Formulation Model.

3.   Identifying Psychic Consequences

a.   Strong emotions
b.   Thoughts/fantasies
c.   Subtle changes in cognition

4.   Coping Mechanisms

a.   Adaptive
b.   Maladaptive

B.   Psychodynamic Formulation

Recurrent difficulties around specific issues (Freudian stage or
Eriksonian crisis)

1.   Dependency (oral stage or basic trust vs. mistrust)
2.   Control (anal stage or autonomy vs. shame and doubt)
3.   Self-esteem (phallic stage or initiative vs. guilt)
4.   Intimacy/triadic relationships (oedipal stage or initiative
        vs. guilt)

C.   Cognitive Perspective

1.   Dysfunctional automatic thoughts
2.   Negative core beliefs
3.   Cognitive distortions

D.   Behavioral Perspective

1.   Is there behavioral reinforcement of a maladaptive behavior?
2.   Is there something that extinguishes a desired behavior?
3.   Is there a paired association between a behavior and an
        environmental cue that initiates the behavior?

(Figure continued)

An Overview of the Biopsychosocial Formulation Model   5

III.   Social Formulation

A.   Creation of a Social Database

1.	Family	6.	Housing
2.	Friends/Significant others	7.	Income
3.	Social issues	8.	Access to health care services
4.	Education	9.	Legal problems/Crime
5.	Work	10.	Other

B.   Assess Social Stressors and Strengths

C.   Perform Cultural and Spiritual Assessments (adapted from DSM-IV)

1.   Cultural/spiritual identity of the patient
2.   Cultural/spiritual explanations of the patient's illness
3.   Cultural/spiritual factors related to the psychosocial environment and levels of functioning
4.   Cultural/spiritual elements of the relationship between the patient and the clinician
5.   Overall cultural/spiritual assessment for diagnosis and treatment

IV.   DSM-IV Differential Diagnosis

V.   Risk Assessment

A.   Create a Risk Assessment Database

1.   Static Risk Factors
2.   Dynamic Risk Factors
3.   Protective Factors
4.   Pathway to Suicide or Violence

(Figure continued)

B.   Formulate a Risk Assessment

1.   Suicide Risk
2.   Violence Risk

C.   Develop a Risk Reduction Plan

1.   Dynamic Risk Factors
2.   Planned Interventions
3.   Status

VI.   Biopsychosocial Treatment Plan

A.   Biological

1.   Recommended Biological Assessments (Reversible Work-Up)

a.   Laboratory studies
b.   Neuroimaging
c.   Other studies

2.   Recommended Biological Interventions

a.   Review and revision of existing medication
b.   Addition of medication
c.   Other somatic treatments

B.   Psychological

1.   Recommended Psychological Assessments

2.   Recommended Psychological Interventions

*(Figure continued)*C.   Social

An Overview of the Biopsychosocial Formulation Model

1. Recommended Social Assessments

3. Recommended Social Interventions

VII. Prognosis

Compliance with treatment
Response to prior treatment
Availability of treatment
Personality/Defense mechanisms
Social Supports

(see Appendix D) is where you will record, organize, and begin the analysis of the data from your patient interview and chart review.

We will review the two initial steps necessary to devise a comprehensive formulation and then demonstrate how the Database Record will be useful to you in organizing this process:

1. The first step is to complete your initial patient interview and chart review utilizing a standard format like the one on the Database Record. Many beginning clinicians feel as though they cannot do a formulation until they have many hours of patient interview data. We discourage this notion. A comprehensive formulation can be initiated after the first interview and will help the clinician focus on pertinent areas of the patient's history in subsequent interviews.

2. The second step is to begin to organize the symptom data you collected into broad areas of psychopathology. We suggest filtering symptoms into eight categories: mood, anxiety, psychosis, somatic, cognitive, substance, personality, and other. In order to perform this step appropriately, you must know the *DSM* categories and the symptoms for each of the disorders in each category. Also, be aware that some symptoms may fit into more

than one category. Feel free to include symptoms in any of the categories in which they may fit. For example, insomnia may be a mood symptom, an anxiety symptom, or the result of a psychotic disorder (in which the patient stays awake at night because of paranoia) or substance-related disorder. Feel free to be overinclusive at this stage.

The Biopsychosocial Formulation Database Record is divided into seven sections. These include the standard Psychiatric History, a Symptom Filter, a Biopsychosocial Formulation section, and sections for Differential Diagnosis, Risk Assessment, Biopsychosocial Treatment Plan, and Prognosis. The Database Record should be used in the following manner:

1. Fill in the Psychiatric History section during or shortly after you conduct your interview with the patient. Remember to review the outline ahead of time so you know what data will be needed for a comprehensive biopsychosocial formulation.

2. Sort specific symptoms as they are reported into the appropriate categories in the Symptom Filter. Individual symptoms should be listed under as many categories as appropriate.

3. After the interview has been concluded, it is time to begin the process of analysis. Complete the Biopsychosocial Formulation section using the data obtained in the first two sections.

Using all the information you elicited, organized, and analyzed, complete the Risk Assessment, Differential Diagnosis, Biopsychosocial Treatment Plan, and Prognosis sections.

Now that you have the bird's-eye view, including a sense of the first two steps in the formulation process and the structure of the Database Record, you are ready to begin formulating. A detailed review of each of the seven major sections of the Biopsychosocial Formulation Model is contained in the ensuing chapters.

2

The Biological Formulation

CREATION OF A BIOLOGICAL/DESCRIPTIVE DATABASE

The biological database will draw upon much of the information you collected in your patient interview and chart review.

Pertinent information for the biological formulation may include the following:

Demographics: Age, race and ethnicity, and gender may influence symptom presentation.

History of present illness: Presenting symptoms analyzed in the Symptom Filter will be crucial for establishing a *DSM* diagnosis.

Past medical history: Physical disorders may cause or exacerbate mental illness.

Medications: Medications may cause or exacerbate mental illness.

Allergies: Rechallenging a patient with a medication, or another medication from the same class, that induced an allergic reaction in the past may result in a life-threatening condition (i.e., anaphylaxis).

Past psychiatric history: This may give clues to the longitudinal course of illness, previous symptoms and diagnoses, and responsiveness to medications.

Substance abuse history: This may be important in establishing comorbid illness or causation of current symptoms.

Family history: This may give clues to genetic predisposition and responsiveness of family members to biological interventions.

Mental status examination: Provides important

information on mood, reality testing, and cognitive status.

Physical and neurological examinations: Abnormalities suggest underlying medical or neurological illness that may cause or exacerbate symptoms.

Diagnostic studies: Abnormalities may suggest underlying medical illness that may cause or exacerbate symptoms.

The first step in developing a biological formulation is to create a biological/descriptive database. As we discussed in the preceding chapter, the Database Record will assist you in eliciting and organizing the requisite clinical data for your formulation. After completing the Database Record, analysis begins by recording symptoms under one or more of the eight categories in the Symptom Filter (Table 2.1).

The Symptom Filter provides a logical means for organizing the information for presentation. It also serves to preclude

Table 2.1   The Eight Categories in the Symptom Filter

Mood

Anxiety

Psychotic

Somatic

Cognitive

Substance

Personality

Other

the inadvertent omission, or "orphaning," of essential data. Individual symptoms should be listed under as many categories as appropriate. The Symptom Filter is a powerful tool that will also facilitate the development of a differential diagnosis and, by applying the principle of parsimony (i.e., Occam's razor), a presumptive "working" diagnosis.

CLINICAL PEARLS

Two useful mnemonics may be employed to guide you in eliciting mood symptoms. The first of these, attributed to Gross (Carlat, 1999), is in the form of a prescription for energy capsules for depression (SIG: E-CAPS) and is used to assess the presence or absence of neurovegetative symptoms (Table 2.2).

The author of the second mnemonic, DIGFAST, is unknown. It is useful for assessing the diagnostic criteria for a hypomanic or manic episode (Table 2.3).

Table 2.2   **SIG: E-CAPS**

S	Sleep disturbance
I	Interest deficit (anhedonia)
G	Guilt (worthlessness, hopelessness)
E	Energy deficit
C	Concentration deficit
A	Appetite disturbance
P	Psychomotor disturbance
S	Suicidal ideation

Table 2.3 DIGFAST

D	Distractibility
I	Indiscretions ("excessive involvement in pleasurable activities")
G	Grandiosity
F	Flight of ideas
A	Activity increase
S	Sleep deficit (decreased need for sleep)
T	Talkativeness (pressured speech)

Once the biological/descriptive data are obtained from the psychiatric interview and medical records and analyzed in the symptom filter, the next step is to determine what biological predispositions and contributing factors are present. This involves considering those biological factors that may have led to the development of the mental disorder. These include genetics, physical conditions, and medications/substances (Table 2.4).

With regard to genetics, it is important to address the presence of mental disorders in the family members of the patient, as most major psychiatric disorders have a genetic predisposition. Physical conditions include medical illnesses, neurological disorders, and nonpathological states such as

Table 2.4 **Biological Predispositions**

Genetics
Physical conditions
Medications/substances

The Biological Formulation

pregnancy. Each physical condition should be evaluated to determine whether the condition could cause or exacerbate the psychiatric disorder. Substances are a very important consideration that is frequently overlooked. These include prescription medications, over-the-counter (OTC) remedies such as cold and allergy preparations and herbal supplements, and alcohol and recreational drugs. When eliciting information about substances, remember to inquire about recent use as well as current use. Substances with long half-lives may continue to exert their effects for substantial periods of time following discontinuation, and patients will rarely feel the need to report substances they are no longer taking.

DO THE DEMOGRAPHICS OF THE PATIENT MATCH THE KNOWN EPIDEMIOLOGY OF THE DISORDER?

When considering various mental disorders as diagnostic possibilities, it is essential that the demographics of the patient (i.e., age, gender, and race) match the known epidemiology of the disorder. For example, it would be unlikely for a patient in his or her sixties to present with new-onset panic disorder in the absence of a general medical condition (e.g., hyperthyroidism) or current or recent substance use (e.g., alcohol or cocaine). So take a few moments to assess whether the demographics of the patient match the known epidemiology of the disorder(s) you have under consideration before you proffer your differential diagnosis (chapter 5).

3

The Psychological Formulation

The psychological formulation is often the most difficult for beginning clinicians. There are many reasons for this. Trainees typically have limited knowledge of the major psychological theories. Moreover, they often believe that a psychological formulation must be based on a specific theory in order to be meaningful. Many clinicians begin their training in busy inpatient units, where the biological and social aspects of care predominate. Even those trainees who may have acquired a basic understanding of one or more psychological theories have limited experience in applying this knowledge in a way that will illuminate a patient's life. Even when senior clinicians articulate psychological formulations, they may not explicate what patient data they utilized in developing their formulations, or their formulations may be so filled with arcane jargon as to be mystifying.

In this chapter, we will provide an overview of what we consider to be the essential elements of a psychological formulation and where you might find the psychological data to support a formulation. We hope to assist beginning clinicians in developing psychological formulations without slavish adherence to a specific psychological theory. Later in the chapter, we will provide an overview of cognitive, behavioral, and psychodynamic theories. This is in no way meant to be an exhaustive treatment of these subjects. Instead, we hope to provide the beginning clinician with sufficient theoretical overview to enhance his or her ability to develop a psychological formulation and to use the formulation to develop a psychologically informed comprehensive treatment plan. Moreover, we strongly believe that a psychological understanding of patients enables clinicians to explicate the genesis of problematic patient behaviors and, in doing so, to help them cope with the difficult feelings that are generated inside them when interacting with certain patients.

As with the biological formulation, the creation of a psychological database that supports the development of a psychological formulation is an important first step. This requires that you complete a psychologically informed patient interview. A social history that focuses solely on meeting developmental milestones (e.g., "The patient began talking at age 1, walked by age 2, began kindergarten at age 4, married at age 20, and divorced at age 32.") will not provide the kind of data necessary to develop a psychological formulation. The following are examples of questions essential for understanding the patient's psychological world (adapted from the Structured Clinical Interview for DSM-IV Axis II Personality Disorders, 1997):

- "What was it like for you growing up?"
- "Who have been the most important people in your life?"
- "Is there anyone you have tried to be like (or not)?"
- "How have you gotten along with other people?"
- "How do you think other people would describe you as a person?"
- "How would you describe yourself as a person?"
- "How do you typically respond to problems or frustrations in life?"

- "Has this caused you problems with anyone? In what ways?"
- "What kinds of things have you done that other people might have found annoying?"
- "What do you admire most in people?"
- "What things do you do that lead to your feeling good about yourself?"
- "If you could change your personality in some ways, how would you want to be different?"

The psychological formulation should provide a story that helps explain (a) how the patient developed certain predisposing psychological vulnerabilities; (b) why these vulnerabilities make current events in the patient's life particularly stressful; (c) what the patient thinks and feels as a result of these stresses; and (d) how the patient attempts to cope with the stress (Table 3.1).

Table 3.1   The Four Components of the Psychological Formulation

Predisposing factors: identification of a psychological theme

Current precipitants: identification of psychosocial stressors

Psychic consequences of current psychosocial stressors: strong emotions and changes in cognition

Dealing with stress: adaptive and maladaptive coping mechanisms

Cognitive, behavioral, and psychodynamic theories each have their own theoretical emphases and terminology for these four components. Nonetheless, if you can learn to think about these components independent of theory and develop a psychological database that covers them, you will be well on your way to developing a cogent psychological formulation. Let us review each of these areas in more detail.

PREDISPOSING FACTORS: IDENTIFICATION OF A PSYCHOLOGICAL THEME

The goal of this component of the formulation is to identify an overarching theme that helps you understand the nature of the vulnerabilities that lead patients to think about themselves, their relationships, and their roles in their environments the way they do.

Although you will become much better at identifying psychological themes as you gain more practice, we suggest you start by attempting to elicit data that point toward one of three common themes that best describes your patient's particular vulnerability (Table 3.2).

What data from your interview and the patient's history might be pertinent to developing a psychological theme? In

Table 3.2   Three Common Psychological Themes

Can I trust others to provide emotional and physical support to me?

Can I remain in control of myself and control my environment?

Can I maintain a healthy sense of self-esteem?

Table 3.3   The Three Types of Patient Data That Are Pertinent to Developing a Psychological Theme

Disruptions in psychological development

Recurrent difficulties in relationships

Revelatory statements and behavior

order to identify this theme, we suggest reviewing three types of patient data (Table 3.3).

Disruptions in Psychological Development

The first component of identifying a theme is to assess for disruptions in psychological development. The clinician should listen carefully for traumatic experiences in the patient's life narrative and identify how the patient coped with those experiences. As noted earlier, this requires that you complete a "psychologically informed" developmental and social history. Listen carefully for discrepancies in the patient's history and do not be afraid to ask clarifying questions when a patient tells you that his childhood was "fine," but later relates that his father was an alcoholic and his mother suffered from recurrent episodes of depression. It would be rare unlikely a person growing up in that environment to have had a "fine" childhood.

To reiterate, focus on eliciting data that point toward one of the three common psychological themes: trust, control, and self-esteem. Were the parents sufficiently available and responsible to provide the patient with emotional and physical support? Were they overly controlling or did they exert so little discipline that the patient felt his environment was constrained or out of control? Did the parents or others belittle the patient so that he or she was unable to develop a healthy sense of self-esteem? Recall that it is the individual's interpretation of the experience that is important, not the clinician's, and that this may involve some degree of distortion of reality. For example, although the perception of rejection, abandonment, and the lack of support by a parent is the result of their unavailability, the reasons for this may be manifold, including postpartum depression, alcohol dependence, or commitments to a career or other children.

These early disruptions are important, as they create expectations in the patient about what interactions with others are likely to be. If these early relationships are disrupted, the patient will enter subsequent relationships (including the relationship with you) believing certain things that may not be true. For example, that they cannot trust and depend on others for support, that others will try to control them, or that others will devalue them.

Recurrent Difficulties in Relationships

The second component of the database in identifying a psychological theme is assessing recurrent difficulties in relationships. What difficulties has the patient had in previous relationships? Did the patient end a relationship because of feelings that the other person was not supportive, was controlling, or devalued the patient in some way? Review past and present relationships, including the patient's relationship with you. Think about what it has been like to work with this patient. Does the patient seem to feel he or she has no responsibility for his or her own care and depends totally on you? Is the patient never on time for appointments and then seems to control what you talk about? Has the patient berated you as "only a student" and not fit to provide care, signaling a need to inflate his or her sense of self-esteem? These peculiarities in your interaction with the patient are likely based on the patient's past relationships with authority figures and so constitute a transference. This is an excellent source of data about the patient. Reviewing past relationships and your relationship with the patient will assist you in predicting the difficulties that will likely arise in the patient's future interactions with others and inform the therapeutic process as these same conflicts continue to unfold in therapy.

Revelatory Statements and Behavior

The third component of the database in identifying a psychological theme is to recognize revelatory statements and behavior. At times, patients will make overtly declarative statements about the themes that are most troublesome for them, such as, "I've learned I can't depend on anyone," "I always end up feeling controlled in relationships," or "I've never been any good at anything." These statements are extremely helpful to you, as they frame the psychological theme in the patient's own words.

The clinician should also listen carefully during the patient's narrative for covert statements that may be equally revelatory. Often, these statements seem odd or inappropriate. For example, a patient relating no emotional response when learning of a spouse's extramarital affair may be struggling with extremely strong emotions about feelings of dependency and trust that were betrayed. Also, listen for what is not being said. An example of this would be when a patient focuses solely on the abusiveness of one parent even though the other parent witnessed the abuse and never intervened on the patient's behalf. This may be relevant to the patient being able to trust that others will be available to help when difficulties in life arise. Careful observation of nonverbal behavior is equally rewarding. For example, a patient, while smiling, relates having injured someone who has tried to control them. Revelatory statements, both overt and covert, and behavior are outstanding sources of data for the psychological formulation. Make every effort to note these in the patient's own words in the Database Record and utilize them in your formulation.

Having reviewed the patient's developmental history, past and current relationships, including the patient's relationship with you, and any revelatory statements or behavior, you should now be able to determine whether the patient seems to have recurring difficulties with any of the three common psychological themes. Frequently, patients will appear to have problems with more than one theme. Keep each theme in mind along with the supporting data. As you work with the patient, you will be able to prioritize which of the areas of difficulty seem most pertinent. Occasionally, especially early on, it may appear that there are no data that point toward one of the common psychological themes. Discussing these cases with a supervisor may be helpful in elucidating the reasons why the identification of a psychological theme seems elusive.

CURRENT PRECIPITANTS: IDENTIFICATION
OF PSYCHOSOCIAL STRESSORS

When a patient presents for psychiatric care, one should always attempt to answer the question, "Why now?" Review the History of Present Illness (HPI) for experiences that either the patient or you believe contributed to the patient presenting for treatment at this time. Try to elucidate the details of what has transpired in the patient's life to cause the current psychosocial stress. If a patient relates that he or she recently lost a job, a sensitive, but detailed, inquiry might reveal additional information that leads to the identification of a common psychological theme. For example, the clinician may learn that the patient became embroiled in a struggle with his boss after the boss refused to allow him to take time off when he wanted to. The patient felt that his boss was overly controlling and became angry, initiated a heated exchange, and was fired. Upon further inquiry, it is learned that the patient's perception of his boss is the result of a longstanding vulnerability of feeling controlled by others based on early childhood experience.

PSYCHOLOGICAL CONSEQUENCES OF CURRENT PSYCHOSOCIAL STRESSORS: STRONG EMOTIONS AND CHANGES IN COGNITION

When patients face psychosocial stressors that have the potential to activate the psychological theme with which they struggle, two categories of psychic consequences may ensue: strong emotions and changes in cognition. The first category of psychic consequences, strong emotions, often includes anxiety and anger. Patients are often keenly aware of the feelings that arise in circumstances that activate their psychological vulnerabilities and present for professional assistance in dealing with these distressing emotions and the maladaptive behavior (e.g., shouting) associated with them. Sometimes, patients may reflexively activate coping mechanisms that prevent them from being aware of these strong emotions. For example, when a patient reports that his wife had an extramarital affair in the absence of an emotional response, the activation of one or more coping mechanisms is highly likely.

The second psychic consequence, changes in cognition, is often more subtle. It is also one that patients are often not as aware of in themselves. In response to a psychosocial stressor activating an underlying psychological vulnerability, patients may experience changes in their views of themselves, others, or their environments. These illogical thoughts and changes in perspective often provide reinforcement to patients about issues related to their psychological themes. For example, in the vignette described in the last section, it may be that the boss merely asked the patient if it would be possible for him to return from vacation one day early in order to be present at an important meeting. Returning might have been easy for the patient because he had not yet finalized his travel plans. Nonetheless, he experienced this logical request as completely unreasonable. We will discuss these changes in cognition, sometimes called automatic dysfunctional thoughts, negative core beliefs, and cognitive distortions, in a later chapter. An assessment for cognitive distortions should be included in every formulation.

DEALING WITH STRESS: ADAPTIVE AND MALADAPTIVE COPING MECHANISMS

In this part of the formulation, you should think about the adaptive and maladaptive mechanisms that patients use to cope with the strong emotions and changes in cognition they are experiencing. Consider all potential coping mechanisms, not just ones that you think are more "psychological." For example, a patient may state that he or she copes with a distressing event by trying to put the issue out of his or her mind or by trying to become distracted by engaging in other activities. The patient may also cope by walking away from an argument, which can be an excellent intervention for someone dealing with anger. Exercise can be a very effective means of coping with feelings of anxiety or anger. Ask patients how they typically deal with problems and frustrations in life. Patients often devise highly adaptive and creative methods for dealing with these issues.

Also, consider the maladaptive coping mechanisms that patients may be utilizing. Here again, patients may use maladaptive coping mechanisms that employ thoughts or actions. For example, a patient may deal with a distressing event by obsessively ruminating for weeks about potential interventions and outcomes, or a patient may engage in hours of fantasy about other activities rather than deal with the problem. Concluding that one can never hold a job because of difficulties with authority figures (i.e., supervisors) would be another example of a maladaptive coping mechanism based on thoughts. On the other hand, binge drinking or cutting oneself to assuage anxiety are examples of maladaptive coping mechanisms based on actions.

We will discuss specific defense mechanisms in a later chapter. A statement about the patient's predominant defense mechanisms and their level of adaptation should be included in most psychological formulations. However, before moving on to a discussion of psychological theories, see if you can remember the four components of the psychological formulation (Table 3.1), the three common psychological themes (Table 3.2), and the three types of patient data that are pertinent to developing a psychological theme (Table 3.3). We believe trainees often lose the basic notion of a psychological formulation because they believe they need to use psychological jargon or employ a specific theoretical construct. Remember, for every patient presentation, the formulation should elucidate the predisposing factors (i.e., the psychological vulnerabilities arising from earlier life experiences that are activated by psychosocial stressors), the current precipitants (i.e., the psychosocial stressors), the psychological consequences of the current psychosocial stressors (i.e., the patient's emotional response, including strong emotions and changes in cognition), and how the patient is dealing with the stress (i.e., what coping mechanisms are being employed, both adaptive and maladaptive). In reviewing the psychological database, consider which theme will have the greatest explanatory power for a given patient (Table 3.2).

Now, we will briefly review some of the psychological theory pertinent to developing psychodynamic, cognitive, and behavioral formulations. This review is meant to demonstrate how a specific psychological theory may, or may not, relate to the formulation structure outlined above and to provide additional information relevant to the psychological formulation. Defense mechanisms (coping mechanisms) that occur in response to psychosocial stressors activating a psychological vulnerability, are especially important to understand and should be considered for inclusion in most psychological formulations. We found the behavioral perspective to be especially helpful in understanding certain disorders, like posttraumatic stress disorder (PTSD) and substance use disorders, and in helping to craft treatment plans that lead to positive reinforcement of adaptive coping mechanisms.

PSYCHODYNAMIC PERSPECTIVE[*]

Sigmund Freud was the first theorist to assert that the difficulties patients encounter in life often have their genesis in childhood experiences and that interactions with early authority figures continue to manifest themselves in the patient's later life. Using more theoretical language, these lifelong psychological themes are referred to as either "conflicts"

---

[*] Adapted from Gabbard, 2005; McWilliams, 1994; Pine, 1990; Sadock and Sadock, 2004; St. Clair, 1999.

or "developmental arrests" that generally arise as the result of either excessive frustration or gratification of the individual's needs during a specific developmental stage.

Freud focused on psychosexual themes while Erik Erikson considered psychosocial themes. They connected each of these themes to psychological disruptions occurring at a specific time (or stage) in the patient's life. The names given to the stages associated with the psychological themes may sound unusual, but they were an attempt to link the psychological issues with the respective biological and social issues the child was struggling with at the time the theme occurred.

It is interesting how often patients who seem to struggle with these themes have had specific psychological insults at the times Freud and Erikson identified. Often, however, our patients have had significant ongoing difficulties throughout their lives, so identifying one specific incident or theme is more difficult. Moreover, according to the principle of over-determination, in understanding the meaning of a problem-atic behavior, one typically finds many contributors, none of which alone would have created the behavior.

Table 3.4 outlines four of the major developmental themes outlined by Freud. You will note that three of the themes are similar to those we emphasized in the basic formulation outline.

Table 3.4   Freud's Major Developmental Themes

Difficulties with trust or having to depend on others
Difficulties with control
Difficulties with self-esteem
Difficulties with triadic relationships (romantic relationships that frequently include a third person)

Erikson proffered an epigenetic model in which an individual must successfully resolve the specific challenge or crisis of one stage in order to move on to the next. Failure to resolve a crisis leads to recurrent difficulties around that specific theme. Look for recurrent difficulties and identify the underlying themes. Table 3.5 outlines the four major developmental themes for consideration and includes the age range associated with the relevant Freudian psychosexual stage and Eriksonian psychosocial crisis.

Freud coined the psychological vulnerability of those who had significant trauma during their childhood a "conflict." He felt that individuals with excessive degrees of unresolved conflict have a tendency to oscillate between positions at the extremes of the theme (e.g., demonstrating submissive, dependent behavior in one instance and overly assertive, totally independent behavior in another) in contrast to "healthier" individuals who behave in a more balanced way.

A second concept that Freud believed was important is that the patient continued to set up circumstances in their

Table 3.5   The Four Major Developmental Themes

Dependency/trust (birth to about 18 months: oral stage or basic trust vs. mistrust)

These people mistrust others or have a tendency to trust people too easily or exhibit both tendencies. They may strive to be totally independent individuals, may become overly dependent upon others or may vary between both behaviors. Difficulties at this phase may result in the development of a dependent personality.

Control (About 18 months to about 3 years: anal stage or autonomy vs. shame and doubt)

These people are excessively controlling, have a tendency to lose control or display both behaviors. They may strive to be obedient, repeatedly defy authority figures or act in both manners. Difficulties at this phase may result in the development of an obsessional personality.

Self-esteem (About 3 to about 5 years: phallic (-oedipal) stage or initiative vs. guilt)

Not having internalized a sense of self-esteem, these people have a tendency to appear grandiose, "narcissistic," cold, or "prickly." They are outspoken, provocative, and seek positions of power and have little internal sense of themselves as worthy individuals. Difficulties in this phase may result in the development of a narcissistic personality.

Difficulties with intimate relationships (About 3 to about 5 years: (phallic-) oedipal stage or initiative vs. guilt)

These individuals may also have a strong tendency to seek out relationships with another person who is already in a relationship (e.g., married or devoted to a parent).

---

life that replayed aspects of the initial psychological trauma. This is why these traumatic experiences continue to manifest themselves throughout the patient's adult life. In technical terms, this is called the *repetition compulsion,* in which an individual unconsciously recreates the circumstances that initially led to the conflict in an effort to gain control and mastery over it. As this scenario plays out, the individual may switch from a historically passive role into an active one, setting up the difficulties that the patient unconsciously wishes to repeat. Look for it whenever you see someone behaving in a way that seems counterproductive.

CREATION OF A PSYCHODYNAMIC DATABASE

The creation of a psychodynamic database will facilitate the development of a psychological formulation from a developmental perspective (Table 3.6). In reviewing this database, consider which theme will have the greatest explanatory power for a given patient.

As you can see, the first three components of the psychodynamic database do not differ, with the exception of noting the developmental stage the patient was in when the trauma occurred. In the *recurrent difficulties in relationships* portion of the database, psychodynamic psychotherapists pay great attention to the relationship between the therapist and the patient

Table 3.6   The Psychodynamic Database

Disruptions in psychological development

Recurrent difficulties in relationships

Revelatory statements and behavior

Current precipitants/psychosocial stressors

Psychic consequences: strong emotions and changes in cognition

Coping mechanisms: thoughts and behavior

Defense mechanisms

as reflecting these early difficulties ("transference" from the patient toward the therapist). You should note any peculiarities in your interaction with the patient, as these are likely to be based on the patient's past relationships with authority figures and so constitute transference. Psychodynamic psychotherapists believe this to be an excellent source of data about the patient. Reviewing past relationships as well as your relationship with the patient will assist you in predicting the difficulties that will likely arise in the patient's future interactions with others and inform the therapeutic process as these same conflicts continue to unfold in therapy. Having reviewed the patient's developmental history, any revelatory statements or behaviors, and the patient's past relationships and current relationships with you, you should determine whether the patient seems to have recurring difficulties with any of the four major developmental themes (Table 3.5).

A major contribution of psychodynamic theory is that it helps us understand the various reflexive and unconscious ways that the patient copes with the strong emotions that arise in response to psychosocial stressors. These coping styles are called defense mechanisms. When a conflict is activated by a precipitant, the patient is often overwhelmed with distressing thoughts or strong feelings of anxiety or anger. Defense mechanisms are mobilized to protect patients against these distressing thoughts and feelings. Understanding which defense mechanisms are being employed may help elucidate the patient's presenting symptoms or illogical aspects of the patient's history.

For example, if the patient who presented for treatment after an argument with his boss had symptoms of depression or irritability, we might consider that the patient was utilizing defenses of introjection (leading to depression) or displacement (leading to irritability) to deal with the angry feelings generated.

Understanding defense mechanisms can be helpful in discerning why clinicians sometimes experience strong feelings when dealing with a particular patient. For example, if a clinician treating a patient begins to experience strong feelings of anger, the patient may be using a defense mechanism known as projective identification (see below). It is essential that clinicians learn to understand defense mechanisms in order to comprehend their own reactions to patients. By doing so, they will be able to maintain a therapeutic stance with patients who have a tendency to induce strongly negative feelings in those who care for them.

Defense mechanisms are generally regarded as being unconscious, that is, the patient is usually unaware that the defense mechanism is being utilized. In most formulations, you should identify the patient's typical response to stressors and assess which defense mechanisms are most frequently mobilized. In a psychodynamic formulation, you should determine the adaptability (i.e., maturity) of the defense mechanisms employed and note whether the patient uses these defenses in an inflexible manner.

We suggest that beginning clinicians become familiar with the defense mechanisms discussed below (adapted from Gabbard, 2005; McWilliams, 1994; Sadock and Sadock, 2004).

Primary (Primitive) Defensive Processes
Acting out
Acting out is expressing an unconscious wish or impulse through action to avoid being conscious of an accompanying affect. The unconscious fantasy is lived out impulsively in behavior, thereby gratifying the impulse, rather than the prohibition against it. Acting out involves chronically giving in to an impulse to avoid the tension that would result from the postponement of expression.

Denial
Denial is a mechanism by which the existence of unpleasant realities is disavowed. The mechanism keeps out of conscious awareness any aspects of external reality that, if acknowledged, would produce anxiety.

Dissociation

Temporarily but drastically modifying a person's character or one's sense of personal identity to avoid emotional distress. Fugue states and hysterical conversion reactions are common manifestations of dissociation. Dissociation may also be found in dissociative identity disorder and the use of pharmacological highs or religious joy.

Introjection

Internalizing the qualities of another person. Although vital to development, introjection serves specific defense functions. When used as a defense, it can obliterate the distinction between the subject and the other person. Through the introjection of a loved other person, the painful awareness of separateness or the threat of loss may be avoided. Introjection of a feared other person serves to avoid anxiety when the aggressive characteristics of the other person are internalized, thus placing the aggression under one's own control. A classic example is identification with the aggressor. Identification with the victim may also take place, whereby the self-punitive qualities of the other person are taken over and established within one's self as a symptom or character trait.

Omnipotent Control

Some feel a compelling need to feel a sense of omnipotent control and to interpret experiences as resulting from one's own unfettered power. If one's personality is organized around seeking and enjoying the sense that one has effectively exercised one's omnipotence, with all other practical and ethical concerns relegated to secondary importance, one can reasonably be construed as being sociopathic (i.e., antisocial). "Getting over on" other people is a central preoccupation and pleasure of individuals whose personalities are dominated by omnipotent control.

Primitive Idealization (and Devaluation)

Viewing other people as either all good or all bad and as unrealistically endowed with great power. Most commonly, the all-good other person is seen as being omnipotent or ideal, and the badness in the all-bad other person is greatly inflated.

Projection

Projection is perceiving and reacting to unacceptable inner impulses and their derivatives as though they were outside the self and were thoughts of others in the patient's life.

Projective Identification

Projective identification is an unconscious three-step process by which aspects of oneself are disavowed and attributed to someone else. The three steps are as follows:

1. The patient projects a feeling state related to another person onto the therapist.

2. The therapist unconsciously identifies with what is projected and begins to feel or behave like the projected feeling state in response to interpersonal pressure exerted by the patient (this aspect of the phenomenon is sometimes referred to as *projective counteridentification*).

3. The projected material is "psychologically processed" and modified by the therapist, who returns it to the patient via reintrojection. The modification of the projected material, in turn, modifies the pattern of interpersonal relatedness.

Splitting

Dividing other people into all-good and all-bad categories, accompanied by the abrupt shifting of other people from one extreme category to the other. Sudden and complete reversals of feelings and conceptualizations about a person may occur. The extreme repetitive oscillation between contradictory self-concepts is another manifestation of the mechanism.

Secondary (Higher-Order) Defensive Processes

Altruism

Altruism is using constructive and instinctually gratifying service to others to undergo a vicarious experience. It includes benign and constructive reaction formation.

Anticipation

Anticipation entails realistically anticipating or planning for future inner discomfort. The mechanism is goal-directed and implies careful planning or worrying and premature but realistic affective anticipation of dire and potentially dreadful outcomes.

Blocking

Blocking is temporarily or transiently inhibiting thinking. Affects and impulses may also be involved. Blocking closely resembles repression but differs in that tension arises when the impulse, affect, or thought is inhibited.

Controlling

Attempting to manage or regulate events or other people in the environment to minimize anxiety and to resolve inner conflicts.

Displacement

Displacement is shifting the focus of an emotion or drive from one idea or person to another that resembles the original in some aspect or quality. Displacement permits the symbolic representation of the original idea or object by one that is less focused or evokes less distress.

Externalization

Externalization is tending to perceive in the external world and in other people elements of one's own personality, including instinctual impulses, conflicts, moods, attitudes, and styles of thinking. Externalization is a more general term than projection.

Humor

Humor is using comedy to overtly express feelings and thoughts without personal discomfort or immobilization and without producing an unpleasant effect on others. It allows the person to tolerate and yet focus on what is too terrible to be borne; it is different from wit, a form of displacement that involves distraction from the affective issue.

Hypochondriasis

Exaggerating or emphasizing an illness for the purpose of evasion and regression. Reproach arising from bereavement, loneliness, or unacceptable aggressive impulses toward others is transformed into self-reproach and complaints of pain, somatic illness, and neurasthenia. In hypochondriasis, responsibility can be avoided, guilt may be circumvented, and instinctual impulses are warded off. Because hypochondria-cal introjects are ego-alien, the afflicted person experiences dysphoria and a sense of affliction.

Identification
Identification is a mechanism by which one patterns oneself after another person. In the process, the self may be permanently altered.

Identification with the Aggressor
In the process of identifying with the aggressor, one incorporates within oneself the mental image of a person who represents a source of frustration. The classic example of the defense occurs toward the end of the phallic-oedipal stage, when a boy, whose main source of love and gratification is his mother, identifies with his father. The father represents the source of frustration, being the powerful rival for the mother. Since the child cannot master or run away from his father, he is obliged to identify with him.

Intellectualization
Excessively using intellectual processes to avoid affective expression or experience. Undue emphasis is focused on the inanimate in order to avoid intimacy with people, attention is paid to external reality to avoid the expression of inner feelings, and stress is excessively placed on irrelevant details to

avoid perceiving the whole. Intellectualization is closely allied to rationalization.

Isolation of Affect

Isolation of affect occurs by splitting or separating an idea from the affect that accompanies it but is repressed.

Passive-Aggressive Behavior

Passive-aggressive behavior is when one expresses aggression toward others indirectly through passivity, masochism, and turning against the self. Manifestations of passive-aggressive behavior include failure and procrastination.

Rationalization

Offering rational explanations in an attempt to justify attitudes, beliefs, or behavior that may otherwise be unacceptable.

Reaction Formation

Transforming an unacceptable impulse into its opposite. Reaction formation is characteristic of obsessional neurosis, but it may occur in other forms of neuroses as well. If this mechanism is frequently used at any early stage of ego development, it can become a permanent character trait, as in an obsessional character.

Regression

In regression, an attempt is made to return to an earlier libidinal phase of functioning to avoid the attention and conflict evoked at the present level of development. It reflects the basic tendency to gain the instinctual gratification of a less-developed period. Regression is a normal phenomenon as well, as a certain amount of regression is essential for relaxation, sleep, and orgasm in sexual intercourse. Regression is also considered an essential concomitant of the creative process.

Repression

Expelling or withholding from consciousness an idea or feeling. Primary repression refers to the curbing of ideas and feelings before they have attained consciousness; secondary repression excludes from awareness what was once experienced at a conscious level. The repressed idea or feeling is not really forgotten in that symbolic behavior may be present. This defense differs from suppression by effecting conscious inhibition of impulses to the point of losing and not just postponing cherished goals. Conscious perception of instincts and feelings is blocked in repression.

Somatization

Somatization is converting psychic derivatives into bodily symptoms and tending to react with somatic manifestations, rather than psychic manifestations.

Sublimation

In sublimation, one achieves impulse gratification and the retention of goals but alters a socially objectionable aim or object to a socially acceptable one. Sublimation allows instincts to be channeled, rather than blocked or diverted. Feelings are acknowledged, modified, and directed toward a significant object or goal, and modest instinctual satisfaction occurs.

Suppression

Suppression occurs when one consciously or semiconsciously postpones attention to a conscious impulse or conflict. Issues may be deliberately cut off, but they are not avoided. Discomfort is acknowledged but minimized.

Clinical Presentations and Defense Mechanisms

Common clinical presentations and their corresponding defense mechanisms are shown in Table 3.7.

Remember that defense mechanisms are coping mechanisms the patient employs to help them deal with strong emotions. As coping mechanisms, defense mechanisms may be either adaptive or maladaptive. Defense mechanisms

Table 3.7   **Common Clinical Presentations and Their Corresponding Defense Mechanisms**

Antisocial personality traits — omnipotent control

Borderline personality traits — splitting, projective identification

Depression — introjection

Irritability — displacement

Impulsive behavior — acting out

Narcissistic personality traits — primitive idealization and devaluation

Paranoia — projection

Unexplained physical symptoms — somatization

can be adaptive in some circumstances and maladaptive in others. For example, in a patient who has recently sustained a myocardial infarction, denial of the seriousness of the illness can be highly adaptive in the acute setting, because the patient could become overwhelmed with anxiety about the consequences of the heart attack. The resultant autonomic response could trigger arrhythmias, extension of the infarction, and death. On the other hand, if denial of the seriousness of the illness continues following discharge from the hospital, the patient may not begin the necessary interventions to reduce further morbidity and mortality from cardiovascular disease, such as dietary changes, moderate exercise, and smoking cessation. As you consider what defense mechanisms your patient is utilizing, try to categorize them as either adaptive or maladaptive.

COGNITIVE PERSPECTIVE*

According to Aaron Beck, the founder of cognitive therapy, our thoughts (i.e., cognitions) directly impact our emotions and behavior. Beck also recognizes the importance of early experiences with authority figures and terms the psychological themes that develop from early experiences "core beliefs." Cognitive therapists recognize the importance of assessing disruptions in psychological development, recurrent difficulties with relationships, and revelatory statements and behavior. In fact, core beliefs are often constructed as revelatory statements. For example, "I'm unable to depend on others," "I can't control myself," and "I'm a nobody." Cognitive therapists are less focused on data from the relationship between the patient and the therapist (the transference and countertransference) than are psychodynamic psychotherapists.

Cognitive therapists are keenly aware of the presence of strong emotions that may result from mental disorders and from psychosocial stressors. A key contribution from cognitive therapy is the observation that mental disorders by themselves, as well as psychosocial stressors, act on psychological vulnerabilities (i.e., core beliefs) to induce subtle, and sometimes not so subtle, cognitive changes in the patient's

---

* Adapted from Beck, 1985; Sadock and Sadock, 2004.

Table 3.8   The Three Components of a Cognitive Formulation

Automatic dysfunctional thoughts

Negative core beliefs

Cognitive distortions (errors in logic)

view of him- or herself and his or her environment. These changes, called "automatic dysfunctional thoughts," "negative core beliefs," and "cognitive distortions" (Table 3.8) may serve to perpetuate or exacerbate the patient's mental disorder. It is important to remember that, in this psychological context, the term "cognitive" refers to the thoughts in an individual's mind, as opposed to "cognitive" in the biological formulation, which refers to the individual's abilities in the domains of attention, concentration, memory, calculation, language, and abstraction.

The first component is automatic dysfunctional thoughts. These are erroneous maladaptive thoughts that occur immediately in response to a trigger (e.g., a perceived slight from someone).

The second component is negative core beliefs. For example, Beck's cognitive triad of depression includes negative views of oneself ("I'm an ineffective person"), the world ("The world is hostile to me"), and the potential for future change ("Things will never change"). Like the psychodynamic theorists, cognitive theorists believe that the automatic dysfunctional thoughts and negative core beliefs may be a consequence of experiences in the patient's early life. You should review the developmental and social history to determine whether you can establish a link between the automatic dysfunctional thoughts, negative core beliefs, and cognitive distortions and the patient's history. If no such link is identifiable, the mental illness itself may be responsible for the changes in the patient's cognitive perspective (e.g., paranoid delusions related to a psychotic disorder).

The third component is cognitive distortions. A cognitive formulation requires identifying the patient's predominant cognitive distortions (errors in logic). We suggest that beginning clinicians become familiar with the common cognitive distortions as described below (adapted from Beck, 1985; Sadock and Sadock, 2004).

Common Cognitive Distortions

All-or-Nothing Thinking

All-or-nothing thinking is also called black-and-white, polarized, or dichotomous thinking. A situation is viewed in only two categories instead of on a continuum. Example: "If I'm not a total success, I'm a failure."

Catastrophizing

Catastrophizing is also called fortune-telling. The future is predicted negatively without considering other, more likely, outcomes. Example: "I'll be so upset, I won't be able to function at all."

Disqualifying or Discounting the Positive

Unreasonably telling yourself that positive experiences, deeds, or qualities do not count. Example: "I did that project well, but that doesn't mean I'm competent; I just got lucky."

Emotional Reasoning

Emotional reasoning is thinking that something must be true because you "feel" (i.e., actually believe) it so strongly, ignoring or discounting evidence to the contrary. Example: "I know I do a lot of things okay at work, but I still feel like I'm a failure."

Labeling

Labeling is putting a fixed, global label on yourself or others without considering that the evidence might more reasonably lead to a less disastrous conclusion. Example: "I'm a loser. He's no good."

Magnification/Minimization

When evaluating yourself, another person, or a situation, you unreasonably magnify the negative and minimize the positive. Example: "Getting a mediocre evaluation proves how inadequate I am. Getting high marks doesn't mean I'm smart."

Mental Filter

A mental filter is also called selective abstraction. It is used when paying undue attention to one negative detail instead of seeing the whole picture. Example: "Because I got one low rating on my evaluation (which also contained several high ratings) it means I'm doing a lousy job."

Mind Reading

Mind reading is believing you know what others are thinking, failing to consider other, more likely, possibilities. Example: "He's thinking that I don't know the first thing about this project."

Overgeneralization

Overgeneralization is making a sweeping negative conclusion that goes far beyond the current situation. Example: [Because I felt uncomfortable at the meeting] "I don't have what it takes to make friends."

Personalization

Personalization is believing others are behaving negatively because of you, without considering more plausible explanations for their behavior. Example: "The repairman was curt to me because I did something wrong."

"Should" and "Must" Statements

"Should" and "must" statements are also called imperatives. This is when you have a precise, fixed idea of how you or others should behave and overestimate the negative consequences of your actions, or those of others, when these expectations are not met. Example: "It's terrible that I made a mistake. I should always do my best."

Tunnel Vision

Tunnel vision is seeing only the negative aspects of a situation. Example: "My son's teacher can't do anything right. He's critical and insensitive and lousy at teaching."

BEHAVIORAL PERSPECTIVE[*]

Learning theory has taught us that behavior, adaptive or maladaptive, can be modified by various factors. The behavior theorists believe that patient vulnerabilities arise through one of two methods. Accordingly, one can use behavioral techniques in the service of the patient. In Skinner's *operant* or *instrumental conditioning*, learning is thought to occur as a result of the *consequences* of one's behaviors and the resultant effect on the environment. *Positive reinforcement* is the process by which certain consequences of the environment increase the probability that

---

[*]   Adapted from Sadock and Sadock, 2004.

the behavior will occur again. Food, water, praise, and money, as well as substances such as opioids, cocaine, and nicotine, all may serve as positive reinforcers. *Negative reinforcement* is the process in which the removal of an aversive event increases the behavior. In this case, any behavior that enables one to avoid or escape a punishing consequence is strengthened. An example would be buckling your seatbelt to turn off the annoying seatbelt alarm in your car. It is important to remember that negative reinforcement is not punishment. *Punishment* is an aversive stimulus (e.g., a slap) that is presented specifically to weaken or suppress an undesired behavior. Punishment reduces the probability that a behavior will occur.

In Pavlov's *classical* or *respondent conditioning*, learning is thought to take place as the result of the *contiguity* of environmental events. That is, when events occur closely together in time, persons will usually come to associate the two. Psychosocial stressors may be associated with previous experiences early in the person's life, thus triggering an emotional or cognitive reaction. Another clinical example of this phenomenon would be a patient being assaulted at the same time a gun is discharged. The patient now reexperiences the assault whenever exposed to a loud noise. The mechanism may suggest how symptoms of posttraumatic stress disorder may be precipitated. Yet another example would be when an individual recovering from cocaine dependence drives through a neighborhood where he or she previously purchased and used drugs. In this scenario, a strong sense of craving is triggered due to the association of the drug use with the environment. *Extinction* occurs when a conditioned stimulus is constantly repeated without the unconditioned stimulus until the response evoked by the conditioned stimulus gradually weakens and eventually disappears.

Although behavioral therapists believe that a particular set of emotions, thoughts, and behaviors can be traced back to childhood, the development of a psychological theme is less important in a behavioral formulation. To understand why a certain maladaptive behavior recurs, the behavioral formulation focuses on three components (Table 3.9).

The first component ("Is there behavioral reinforcement of a maladaptive behavior?") relates to operant conditioning. The second component ("Is there something that extinguishes a desired behavior?") and the third component ("Is there a paired association between a behavior and an environmental cue that initiates the behavior?") relate to classical conditioning.

Table 3.9   **The Three Components of a Behavioral Formulation**

Is there behavioral reinforcement of a maladaptive behavior?

Is there something that extinguishes a desired behavior?

Is there a paired association between a behavior and an environmental cue that initiates the behavior?

4

The Social Formulation

CREATION OF A SOCIAL DATABASE

Clinicians are interested in a patient's social life because
there are abundant data demonstrating that patients sub-
jected to acute and chronic social stressors are more likely

to develop, or have more frequent exacerbations of their, psychiatric conditions. The social formulation assesses the patient's social strengths and vulnerabilities in order to consider social interventions that might reduce the stress the patient is under.

As with the biological and psychological formulations, the first step in developing a social formulation is the creation of a social database. The 10 categories for the social database are adapted from the *DSM-IV* (2000) (Table 4.1). The creation of a social database is accomplished by assessing the patient's current level of functioning in each of the categories. Regrettably, clinicians often focus only on the patient's limitations. A proper social formulation also considers the patient's social strengths.

The first category is *family*. Stressors might include the death of a family member; health problems in the family; disruption of the family by separation, divorce, or estrangement; removal from the home; remarriage of a parent; emotional, physical, or sexual abuse; parental overprotection; neglect of a child; inadequate discipline; discord with siblings; and birth of a sibling.

The second category is *friends/significant others*. Stressors might include the death or loss of a friend or significant other.

Table 4.1   **The Ten Categories for the Social Database**

Family

Friends/significant others

Social environment

Education

Work

Housing

Income

Access to healthcare services

Legal problems/crime

Other

The third category is *social environment*. Stressors might include inadequate social support; living alone; difficulty with acculturation; discrimination; and adjustment to a life-cycle transition, such as retirement.

The fourth category is *education*. Stressors might include illiteracy, academic problems, discord with teachers or classmates, and an inadequate school environment.

The fifth category is *work*. Stressors might include unemployment, threat of a job loss, stressful work schedule, difficult work conditions, job dissatisfaction, job change, and discord with the boss or coworkers.

The sixth category is *housing*. Stressors might include homelessness, inadequate housing, an unsafe neighborhood, and discord with neighbors or landlord.

The seventh category is *income*. Stressors might include extreme poverty, inadequate finances, and insufficient welfare support.

The eighth category is *access to health care services*. Stressors might include inadequate health-care services, unavailability of transportation to health-care facilities, and inadequate health insurance.

The ninth category is *legal problems/crime*. Stressors might include arrest, incarceration, litigation, and being the victim of a crime.

The tenth category is *other*. Stressors might include exposure to disasters, war, or other hostilities; discord with nonfamily caregivers such as a counselor, social worker, or physician; and unavailability of social service agencies.

PERFORM CULTURAL AND SPIRITUAL ASSESSMENTS

The cultural assessment is designed to assist the clinician in evaluating and reporting the impact of a patient's culture on the patient's clinical presentation. It provides a systematic review of the patient's cultural background, the role of their culture in the expression and evaluation of symptoms and dysfunction, and the effect that differences in culture may have on the relationship between the patient and the clinician.

The outline for the cultural assessment is meant to supplement the multiaxial diagnostic assessment and to address difficulties that may be encountered in applying *DSM-IV* criteria in a diverse cultural environment.

Spirituality and religious beliefs are a major focus of many patients' lives. Accordingly, the spiritual assessment is a key component of the social formulation. The approach to the spiritual assessment is analogous to that of the cultural assessment. The categories are adapted from those in the *DSM-IV* (1994) (Table 4.2).

The first category is the *cultural and spiritual identity of the patient*. Note the patient's ethnic or cultural reference groups. For immigrants and ethnic minorities, note separately the degree of involvement with both the culture of origin and the host culture. Also note language abilities, use, and preference, including multilingualism. Note the patient's spiritual reference group, the degree of involvement in spiritual

Table 4.2   Categories for the Cultural and Spiritual Assessment

Cultural and spiritual identity of the patient

Cultural and spiritual explanations of the patient's illness

Cultural and spiritual factors related to the psychosocial environment and levels of functioning

Cultural and spiritual elements of the relationship between the patient and the clinician

Overall cultural and spiritual assessment for diagnosis and treatment activities, and the impact that the patient's spirituality has on his or her life.

The second category is *cultural and spiritual explanations of the patient's illness*. Identify the predominant idioms of distress through which symptoms or the need for social support are communicated (e.g., "nerves," possessing spirits, somatic complaints, inexplicable misfortune), the meaning and perceived severity of the patient's symptoms in relation to norms of the cultural reference group, any local illness category used by the patient's family and community to identify the condition (i.e., culture-bound syndromes), the perceived causes or explanatory models that the individual and the reference group use to explain the illness, and current preferences for and past experiences with professional and popular sources of care. Identify the perceived causes or explanatory models that the patient and reference group use to explain the illness (e.g., punishment for sin), the meaning and perceived severity of the patient's symptoms in relation to norms of the spiritual reference group (e.g., sanctification through suffering), any local illness category used by the patient's family and spiritual reference group to identify the condition (e.g., demonic possession), and current preferences for and past experiences with representatives of their faith as well as secular sources of care.

The third category is *cultural and spiritual factors related to the psychosocial environment and levels of functioning*. Note culturally relevant interpretations of social stressors, available social supports, and levels of functioning and disability. This would include stresses in the local social environment and the role of religion and kin networks in providing emotional, instrumental, and informational support. Note spiritually relevant interpretations of social stressors, available social supports, and levels of functioning and disability. This includes stresses in the local social environment and the role of spiritual and kin networks in providing emotional, instrumental, and informational support.

The fourth category is *cultural and spiritual elements of the relationship between the patient and the clinician*. Indicate differences in culture and social status between the patient and the clinician and problems that these differences may cause in diagnosis and treatment (e.g., difficulty in communicating in the individual's first language, in eliciting symptoms or understanding their cultural significance, in negotiating an appropriate relationship or level of intimacy, in determining whether a behavior is normative or pathological). Indicate differences in spiritual beliefs between the patient and the clinician and problems that these differences may cause in diagnosis and treatment. This includes difficulty in communicating with the patient in a spiritually relevant manner, in eliciting symptoms or understanding their spiritual significance, in negotiating an appropriate relationship or level of intimacy, and in determining whether a behavior is normative or pathological.

The fifth category is the *overall cultural and spiritual assessment for diagnosis and treatment*. The formulation concludes with a discussion of how cultural and spiritual considerations specifically influence comprehensive diagnosis and treatment. For example, disparate cultural and spiritual backgrounds in the patient and clinician may impact a number of key variables that will ultimately determine whether treatment is successful. Some of these are listed in Table 4.3.

Table 4.3 Key Variables in Determining the Success of Treatment When Cultural and Spiritual Backgrounds Between the Patient and Clinician Differ

Diagnosis: Are the symptoms explained on the basis of the patient's cultural and spiritual background or do they have a bona fide mental disorder?

Acceptance of diagnosis: How stigmatizing is the acceptance of a mental disorder?

Compliance with treatment: What meaning does the recommended treatment have for the patient?

Therapeutic alliance: Will the patient be able to trust someone from a different cultural and spiritual background?

5

Differential Diagnosis

After completing the Database Record, using the Symptom Filter to sort the presenting symptoms into eight major categories, and noting the presence of potential biological, psychological, and social predispositions to psychiatric disorders, the next step in developing the overall formulation is to construct a multiaxial *DSM-IV* (2000) differential diagnosis using the Database Record as a guide. The differential diagnosis is the list of potential *DSM-IV* diagnoses the patient may have. The importance of developing a comprehensive, but not overly inclusive, differential diagnosis cannot be overemphasized.

Using the Symptom Filter as a guide, work through each of the eight categories, constructing a set of *DSM-IV* diagnoses based on the symptom profile you constructed. Until you become familiar with the symptom criteria for the *DSM-IV* disorders, this step will be a laborious process. However, once you become familiar with the symptom profile defining each disorder, this process will be straightforward.

You may have a lengthy list of potential disorders at the outset. Identify those diagnoses you are certain the patient has by designating them as "presumptive diagnoses" ("working diagnoses"). Identify those diagnoses which you are less certain of, or need additional data to determine whether they are present, by designating them as "rule-out diagnoses" (meaning that over time you expect to either include — "rule them in" — or exclude — "rule them out" — them as diagnoses).

After completing your set of possible *DSM-IV* diagnoses, review the biological, psychological, and social predispositions to assist you in prioritizing the differential diagnosis. For example, the family history may suggest whether one of the diagnoses you are considering is more likely than another. If the patient's mother has bipolar disorder, but the patient is now presenting with major depression, it would be reasonable to include a "rule out" for bipolar disorder in your differential diagnosis.

As we discussed, physical conditions, medications, and substances may cause or exacerbate the patient's presenting symptoms. Using a standard text, review the patient's principal diagnoses to determine whether any physical condition, medication, or substance may be contributing to the patient's presenting symptoms. If you suspect there may be a contributing factor, designate this using the appropriate *DSM-IV* diagnostic criteria (i.e., *Mood Disorder Due to Hypothyroidism*) and list this as a rule-out diagnosis. As you begin to develop your differential diagnosis, the process will again seem laborious, as it requires that you review and cross-reference all of the patient's biological, psychological, and social contributors with your diagnoses. However, over time, you will begin to recognize common factors that contribute to the patient's clinical presentation. Your ability to recognize these factors and utilize this knowledge in constructing a differential diagnosis, risk assessment, treatment plan, and prognosis will set you apart from other clinicians. The time spent is well worth it.

Two common errors must be assiduously avoided when developing a differential diagnosis. The first is failing to account for all of the data obtained from the psychiatric interview (i.e., "orphaning" data). The second common error is failing to develop as broad a differential diagnosis as the data will support. With respect to the second error, "shotgun" approaches to differential diagnosis are equally problematic. Any diagnosis you include in your list must be supported by the data. Study the differential diagnosis sections for the more common mental disorders in *DSM-IV* and construct a list of possibilities, in decreasing order of probability, after each patient evaluation until it becomes second nature. This is one of the skill sets that differentiate the average clinician from the exceptional one.

Once a differential diagnosis is constructed, it will be necessary to identify one or more presumptive or "working" diagnoses to direct your interventions. Avoid the frequently strong temptation to prematurely narrow the differential diagnosis by jumping immediately to a presumptive diagnosis. This is one of the most common, and potentially costly (for both you and the patient), errors in clinical practice. Do not relax on this one. Your reputation, and the patient's well-being, may depend on it.

6

Risk Assessment

The assessment of whether a patient is at risk of harming him- or herself or others is a critical component of the overall formulation. The risk assessment is based on one's knowledge of the biological, psychological, and social risk factors. Therefore, the risk assessment is only considered once the biological, psychological, and social formulations and the differential diagnosis are completed. The risk assessment addresses two related issues: the patient's potential for self-harm (suicidality) and their potential for violence toward others. Demographic and other risk factors are useful guides in assessing risk. However, it is important to remember that these risk factors, by themselves, do not accurately predict risk in a specific patient. That is why clinical judgment is so important. A final point to keep in mind is that risk factors are not equivalent. For example, two patients may have four risk factors each. However, a depressed woman with a chronic physical illness, no social supports, and a 90-day supply of amitriptyline poses a far greater suicide risk than an elderly widower with a chronic physical illness who lives alone and has no readily available lethal means at his disposal.

RISK FACTORS FOR SUICIDE

A useful mnemonic that summarizes the major risk factors for suicide is SAD PERSONAS (Table 6.1). This is Campbell's adaptation of Patterson's SAD PERSONS scale (Campbell, 2004 ; Patterson, 1983):

S — Sex. Remember that women attempt suicide more often than men, but men complete suicide more often than women.

A — Age. Keep in mind that there is a bimodal distribution of increased risk for suicide in adolescents and the elderly.

D — Depression. However, this refers to any serious mental disorder.

P — Previous attempt. Past behavior is always the best predictor of future behavior. Accordingly, a history of attempted suicide is a major risk factor for current suicide.

E — Ethanol abuse. This category also includes other substances that cause disinhibition and impaired judgment.

R — Rational thought loss. This refers to any significant cognitive impairment, irrespective of the etiology (e.g., dementia or psychosis).

S — Social supports lacking. This refers to limited social supports.

O — Organized plan.

N — No spouse.

A — Availability of lethal means. This includes firearms, stockpiled medication, and poisons.

S — Sickness. This refers to significant, usually chronic, physical illness.

Table 6.1 The SAD PERSONAS Mnemonic for Risk Factors for Suicide

S	Sex
A	Age
D	Depression
P	Previous attempt
E	Ethanol abuse
R	Rational thought loss
S	Social supports lacking
O	Organized plan
N	No spouse
A	Availability of lethal means
S	Sickness

RISK FACTORS FOR VIOLENCE

With regard to the risk assessment for violence, three categories of risk factors are considered: patient-related, historical, and environmental. These are summarized in Table 6.2.

APPROACH TO RISK ASSESSMENT

Our approach to risk assessment mirrors that of the biological, psychological, and social formulations. The first step is to create a database, the second step is to formulate the risk assessment, and the third step is to develop a risk reduction (i.e., treatment) plan. This is outlined in Figure 6.1 and Table 6.3.

```
┌─────────────────────────────────────────────────────┐
│                                                     │
│         Create a Risk Assessment Database           │
│                       ↓                             │
│         Formulate the Risk Assessment               │
│                       ↓                             │
│         Develop a Risk Reduction Plan               │
│                                                     │
└─────────────────────────────────────────────────────┘
```

Figure 6.1   **The risk assessment flowchart.**

Table 6.2   Risk Factors for Violence

Patient-related risk factors

Age (adolescents and young adults)

Sex (males > females)

Socioeconomic status (the lower, the more violence)

Intelligence (the lower, the more violence)

Education (the more limited, the more violence)

Certain psychiatric disorders (e.g., dysphoric mania, paranoid psychosis, substance intoxication, severe personality disorder with difficulty controlling anger, impulsivity, or antisocial behavior)

Certain neurologic disorders (e.g., frontal lobe injury)

Progressive psychomotor agitation

Historical risk factors

Violence or criminal arrests

Childhood abuse

Employment instability

Residential instability

Environmental risk factors

Discharge to same location where the most recent conflict arose

Environment with increased social control or increased social strain

Limited social supports

Availability of substances

Availability of weapons

Table 6.3   **Approach to Risk Assessment**

Create a risk assessment database

Static risk factors

Dynamic risk factors

Protective factors

Pathway to suicide or violence

Formulate the risk assessment

Suicide risk

Violence risk

Develop a risk reduction plan

Dynamic risk factors

Planned interventions

Status

Step 1: Create a Risk Assessment Database

Static risk factors are not subject to change by intervention and are typically historical; examples include demographic information and a prior history of suicide or violence.

Dynamic risk factors are subject to change by intervention or treatment or control of the situation and are typically current; examples include medication nonadherence and access to firearms.

Protective factors mitigate the risk of following through with the idea or planned action; examples include dependent children and religious beliefs against suicide and violence.

Pathway to suicide or violence represents the sequential steps in a process that culminates in suicide or violence (Figure 6.2).

Step 2: Formulate the Risk Assessment

It is important to consider both the pathway and the context when formulating a risk assessment. The more steps there are in the pathway (i.e., predatory vs. affective violence), the greater the opportunity to explore the issues and intervene.

Suicide	Affective Violence	Predatory Violence
Idea	Grievance	Grievance
↓	↓	↓
Research/Planning	Idea/Emotion	Idea
↓	↓	↓
Preparation	Attack	Research/Planning
↓		↓
Suicidal Act		Preparation
		↓
		Breach of Barrier
		↓
		Attack

Figure 6.2   Pathways to suicide and violence.

Assess how far along the pathway the person has progressed. The farther along the pathway, the greater the likelihood they have of carrying out the suicidal act or attack. Also, look for boundary crossings (i.e., passing a point of no return), such as purchasing a handgun, which commit the person to a level or course of action.

The risk assessment is context dependent: the more imminent the suicide or violence, the less important the static risk factors. Consider the setting in which the risk assessment takes place (i.e., outpatient setting, emergency department, or inpatient unit).

All expressions of suicidal ideation should initially be taken seriously. However, keep in mind that certain individuals express suicidal intent as a means of meeting their psychological or material needs (e.g., attention and concern from others or room and board, respectively). It is only following a thorough evaluation that factitious disorder and malingering can be distinguished from real suicidal ideation. Moreover, prior expressions of malingered suicidal ideation do not eliminate the possibility of real suicidal ideation in the present.

Two types of violence risk should be considered:

Affective ("hot") violence: The result of internal and external stimuli that evoke an intense and patterned activation of the autonomic nervous system, accompanied by threatening vocalizations and attacking or defending postures; associated with foreshadowing behaviors.

Predatory ("cold") violence: Planned, purposeful, goal-directed; unlike affective violence, is not reactive and requires emotional detachment; the hallmark of the psychopathic character; more dangerous behavior, as there are no behaviors that foreshadow it.

Step 3: Develop a Risk Reduction Plan

- Addressing dynamic risk factors can mitigate risk. It is helpful to construct a table listing each of the dynamic risk factors, the planned intervention, and the status of the intervention as depicted in Table 6.4.

- Hospitalization, voluntary or involuntary, is the most effective means of preempting imminent suicide or violence.

- With regard to violent intent against an identifiable person, "target hardening" may also be employed. Specific approaches include issuing a Tarasoff warning to the police and the potential victim and, if feasible, advising the potential victim to relocate to another geographic area.

Table 6.4   Sample Risk Reduction Plan

DYNAMIC RISK FACTORS	PLANNED INTERVENTIONS	STATUS
Psychosis/medication nonadherence	Depot antipsychotic	Receiving medication
Alcohol and cocaine abuse	Drug rehabilitation program/ random urine drug screening	Refused
Access to firearms	Removal of firearms from the home	Removed and stored
Living with verbally abusive relative	Relocation to supported housing	In progress

7

The Biopsychosocial Treatment Plan

The next step involves the development of a comprehensive biopsychosocial treatment plan. The biopsychosocial formulation, differential diagnosis, and risk assessment will be immensely helpful in informing the treatment plan for your patient. The treatment plan is divided into three sections (biological, psychological, and social) with two components in each section (assessment and interventions).

THE BIOLOGICAL TREATMENT PLAN

Biological Assessment: Recommended Reversible Workup

The "reversible" workup ensures that the patient does not have a physical condition or take any medications/substances that, if addressed (or "reversed"), might improve the patient's psychiatric condition. Begin by using a standard textbook of psychiatry to identify potential underlying medical conditions, and the diagnostic studies necessary to confirm these, that could be causing or exacerbating the patient's psychiatric condition. Be sure to include studies that ensure that any predisposing medical condition you have already identified is adequately treated. The reversible workup can be divided into three areas of concentration as shown in Table 7.1.

Laboratory Studies

Consult a standard textbook of psychiatry to see which laboratory studies are pertinent for the differential diagnosis you have. Routine laboratory studies for almost all patients should include a complete blood count (CBC); serum chemistries (electrolytes, glucose, blood urea nitrogen [BUN], creatinine,

Table 7.1   The "Reversible" Workup

Laboratory studies
Imaging studies
Other studies

magnesium, calcium, phosphate); liver function tests [LFTs]), TSH (thyroid-stimulating hormone), folate, and vitamin B_{12} levels; rapid plasma reagin (RPR) or Venereal Disease Research Laboratory (VDRL) test for syphilis; urinalysis; urine toxicology screen; and relevant medication levels (e.g., lithium and valproic acid). A urine pregnancy test should also be obtained in women of childbearing age. Special laboratory studies should be ordered only if clinically indicated (e.g., hepatitis screen, human immunodeficiency virus [HIV] ELISA, or Lyme ELISA in high-risk patients).

Imaging Studies

A standard chest X-ray may be clinically indicated in selected patients (e.g., in the presence of a fever or cough). Neuroimaging studies are expensive and time consuming to obtain. Accordingly, they should never be ordered without careful consideration of their clinical indication. Review the mental status examination, the physical examination, and, especially, the neurological examination carefully to determine if there are any findings that would suggest an underlying neurological condition that might be elucidated by neuroimaging.

The two most frequently ordered neuroimaging studies are cranial computed axial tomography (CT scan) and brain magnetic resonance imaging (MRI). Remember that a CT scan is indicated for suspected acute intracranial hemorrhage (e.g., head injury or acute stroke) and is better than an MRI at detecting intracranial calcifications. It is also used when an MRI is contraindicated (e.g., in patients with pacemakers, cochlear implants, or magnetic surgical clips). MRI is the preferred procedure for all other indications, including a desire to avoid ionizing radiation (e.g., pregnancy). Functional neuroimaging, such as positron-emission tomography (PET), single photon-emission computed tomography (SPECT), and functional MRI (fMRI), is used primarily for research purposes but will likely have greater clinical application in the future.

Other Studies

The category labeled *other studies* includes neurophysiological studies (e.g., electroencephalography [EEG] to detect seizure disorders, polysomnography to assess sleep physiology), neuropsychological testing (to assess cognitive deficits), and biologically based diagnostic rating scales (e.g., Abnormal Involuntary Movement Scale [AIMS] to assess for tardive dyskinesia, a side effect of antipsychotic medications, and AUDIT questionnaire to further assess alcohol abuse).

Biological Interventions — Somatic Treatment

The next step is to decide what somatic treatment you will order (Table 7.2). For beginning clinicians, this step

Table 7.2 **Somatic Treatment**

Review and revision of existing medications

Addition of medication

Other somatic treatments

---

is frequently taken without the important, but more time-consuming, assessment of current physical conditions and medication. It is essential to ensure that the patient's current physical conditions are being optimally managed and that the patient's current medication regimen is carefully reviewed to determine whether each medication is necessary (remember, we live in an age of polypharmacy) and whether the dose of the medication is appropriate.

Begin by reviewing and, if necessary, revising the existing medication regimen in consultation with the primary care provider caring for the patient. Carefully review all current and recently discontinued medications (recall that many medications have long half-lives with clinical effects lasting for significant periods of time following discontinuation), and consider either reducing the doses of, or discontinuing, current medications that may be contributing to the mental disorder (e.g., lipophilic beta blockers, such as propranolol, in a patient with a depressive disorder).

Next, consider the addition of psychotropic medication. Remember to optimize the dose of any current medications before adding another medication or utilizing augmentation strategies. Before adding a medication, it is important to conduct a "risk–benefit analysis." What risks might accrue to the patient from the medication? Consider risks like common side effects, known medication interactions, and uncommon side effects that might be particularly dangerous in your patient. Consider benefits like the seriousness of the presenting symptoms, the likelihood that the medication will be effective for the treatment of the psychiatric disorder, and whether the medication might have additional benefits (i.e., bupropion in a patient with depression who also smokes cigarettes). Do the same risk–benefit analysis for each of the psychotropic medications you are considering for the patient before you decide which medication you will be recommending to the patient.

Prescribing clinicians should consider pharmacokinetic and pharmacodynamic factors such as protein binding (highly protein-bound psychotropic medications may result in displacement of other highly protein-bound drugs such as aspirin, digoxin, furosemide, theophylline, and warfarin), cytochrome P450 enzyme inhibition or induction, drug interactions, and side effects. All clinicians should know the dosing schedule and side effects, both common and serious, for each medication their patient is taking.

The category labeled *other somatic treatments* includes electroconvulsive therapy (ECT), light therapy, and treatments such as repetitive transcranial magnetic stimulation (rTMS), vagal nerve stimulation (VNS), and deep brain stimulation (DBS).

Always remember that obtaining informed consent from the patient or, when appropriate, the patient's guardian must be completed before instituting somatic treatments. Proper informed consent requires knowledge (i.e., information on the risks and benefits of the intervention), voluntariness (i.e., the patient is not subject to coercion), and competence (i.e., the patient must demonstrate a factual and rational understanding of the information provided). The requisite disclosure of information includes the patient's diagnosis, the therapeutic alternatives (including no treatment), and the risks and benefits of the specific treatments (including no treatment). If you have concerns about the patient's ability to provide informed consent, you should note that in your formulation.

THE PSYCHOLOGICAL TREATMENT PLAN

Psychological Assessment

Psychological testing may be utilized to assess current symptom severity or to provide additional data about the patient's

underlying condition. These tests include self-adminis-
tered and clinician-administered psychologically based rating scales. Psychometric scales like the Beck Depression
Inventory (BDI), Yale–Brown Obsessive-Compulsive Scale
(Y-BOCS), and Brief Psychiatric Rating Scale (BPRS) are
used to determine current symptom severity of depression,
obsessions/compulsions, and psychosis, respectively. They are
usually used at the initial assessment and then periodically
thereafter to determine how well the patient is responding to
treatment. Other forms of psychological testing include projective testing (e.g., Rorschach, Thematic Apperception Test
[TAT]) and personality testing (e.g., Minnesota Multiphasic
Personality Inventory [MMPI-2], Millon Clinical Multiaxial
Inventory [MCMI-III]). Biologically based rating scales (e.g.,
AIMS) and neuropsychological testing (e.g., Halsted–Reitan
neuropsychological battery) were listed in this chapter in
the biological assessment under "Other Studies" as they are
employed to assess biological issues (i.e., cognitive deficits).

Psychological Interventions

The psychological formulation you constructed provides an
extremely helpful guide to utilize in developing your psychological treatment plan. Remember, your psychological formulation had four components:

1. The patient's psychological vulnerabilities, manifested in one or more psychological themes
2. The current precipitants psychosocial stressors
3. The psychic consequences of the psychosocial stressors, including strong emotions and changes in cognition
4. The patient's coping mechanisms, both adaptive and maladaptive

By considering each of these areas, clinicians have an opportunity to improve the patient's psychological health and clinical outcome.

Let us review each of these four components in some detail in order to provide an overview of how a psychotherapist might intervene to help the patient. This brief review of potential interventions in each of the four components will also compare and contrast psychological treatment interventions from both cognitive-behavioral therapy (CBT) and psychodynamic psychotherapy (PDP) perspectives. As previously stated, we erred on the side of oversimplification in order to make these concepts as accessible to trainees as is possible.

The Patient's Psychological Vulnerabilities

Patients are often unaware of their psychological vulnerabilities and so feel baffled by the recurrent difficulties they experience in their lives. Having a conscious understanding of their psychological vulnerabilities gives patients hope that they will be able to manage these vulnerabilities and so decreases their distress.

Both CBT and PDP approaches provide opportunities to diminish the patient's psychological vulnerabilities by making the patient more consciously aware of the themes with which they struggle. In a CBT-oriented therapy, the patient and therapist explicitly work to determine what core beliefs the patient has about him- or herself and his or her environment. In a PDP therapy, the process is less explicit, but as the therapist and patient review present and past issues, and as the patient talks about his or her experience to the therapist, the patient develops a conscious understanding of psychological vulnerabilities. In both forms of psychological treatment, the patient developing a conscious understanding of his or her psychological vulnerabilities is seen as a necessary step in reducing distress.

The Current Precipitants Psychosocial Stressors

Helping the patient identify which psychosocial stressors they are particularly vulnerable to and reducing the current psychosocial stressors are two methods to help diminish their distress.

CBT therapists explicitly attempt to identify situations that trigger the patient's distress and help the patient prepare and rehearse methods to mitigate the effect of the psychosocial stressor. PDP therapists are less likely to be explicit about identifying triggers or crafting methods to mitigate the effects of the stressor; however, by focusing attention on potential similarities between current and past issues, as well as by paying attention to what stress in the relationship between the patient and the therapist caused a similar reaction in the patient, the patient gradually becomes aware of the psychosocial stressors to which he or she is vulnerable.

Psychic Consequences of the Psychosocial Stressors

As a result of the stress they are under, patients may have strong emotional reactions, thoughts, and fantasies about the issue, and subtle cognitive changes. Becoming consciously aware of these strong emotions, the content of their thoughts, and the presence of the cognitive distortions can be quite helpful for patients, as it allows them to consider more adaptive coping mechanisms to deal with these psychic consequences.

CBT and PDP therapists explicitly attempt to identify these strong emotions engendered by these stressors. While CBT therapists are generally focused on overt emotional reactions (such as anxiety or anger), PDP therapists focus on both overt feelings as well as feelings the patient may not be consciously aware of having.

CBT therapists focus more on identifying the cognitive processing errors of the patient, while PDP therapists focus more on the content of the patient's thoughts and fantasies about the stress.

The Patient's Coping Mechanisms

Improving adaptive coping mechanisms and minimizing maladaptive coping mechanisms are two extremely important methods of helping a patient decrease distress. Helping the patient to understand his or her own adaptive and maladaptive coping mechanisms is a first step in the process. However, most psychotherapists hope that the patient will develop an understanding of new adaptive coping mechanisms during the course of therapy.

Both CBT and PDP attempt to provide patients with improved ability to cope with the situations they are facing. However, CBT and PDP have relatively divergent mechanisms for reaching this common goal. It is important to note that many therapists utilize elements from both CBT and PDP therapies in their work with patients. This eclectic approach allows therapists to tailor their approaches to the specific difficulties with which a patient is presenting.

Cognitive Behavioral Psychotherapy CBT attempts to provide the patient with a set of tools with which to manage the strong emotions and subtle cognitive changes encountered. Having overtly identified vulnerabilities and the circumstances under which the vulnerabilities are activated (psychosocial stressors), the patient and CBT therapist set out to develop a plan to manage the strong emotions and correct the distorted cognitions. Using this plan, CBT therapists encourage the patient to test the plan by exposing themselves to the situations that cause difficulty, and so reinforce the skills the patient learned through the positive reinforcement of a good outcome. Anger management and assertiveness training, relaxation training to decrease anxiety, identifying and avoiding/coping with triggers for substance abuse, and social skills training to improve a patient's ability to read other's social cues and respond appropriately are all examples of CBT-oriented treatments.

CBT therapists may also counsel patients to do activities that may reinforce a desired feeling state. For example, a patient who feels anxious may benefit from going to the gym and getting exercise. A patient who is depressed may benefit by asking a friend to go to the movies. These less complicated behavior interventions that provide reinforcement of a desired mood or behavior should not be overlooked as "too simple."

Patients can often benefit from these simple interventions given as homework between sessions. You should also remember to reinforce adaptive cognitive and behavioral coping mechanisms that the patient may already be employing.

CBT Treatment Example A CBT therapist may counsel the patient who became angry when his boss asked him to change his vacation plans to identify the emotion of becoming angry and to politely excuse himself from the situation. The therapist may then suggest taking a walk or doing some relaxation exercises that would decrease the patient's strong emotions (anger management). The therapist may inform the patient that he has a tendency not to fully understand issues when angry (due to cognitive distortions) and so have the patient go back to the boss at a time when he is relaxed in order to understand the boss's request more fully. The therapist might counsel the patient not to make a decision until he has had time to think through the request, perhaps with the aid of the therapist. Finally, the therapist may suggest methods for responding to the boss's request (i.e., through writing) that may reduce the likelihood of an unpleasant interaction.

Psychodynamic Psychotherapy In PDP therapy, there is less focus on providing the patient with a set of methods to manage the strong emotions and cognitive sequelae of the psychosocial stress. In fact, providing these suggestions is somewhat contraindicated, as it would interfere with the patient's development of a set of thoughts and feelings (the transference that is relatively independent of actual events in the therapy). Instead, in PDP, the therapeutic goal is to allow the patient to understand his or her vulnerabilities, to become conscious of and more comfortable with having these strong feelings and cognitions/fantasies, and to be able to express them directly to the therapist. By expressing him- or herself directly, the patient will not need to use unconscious, often maladaptive defense mechanisms like displacement, denial, or projection, to cope with the strong feelings and thoughts. The patient will be able to have conscious access to the strong emotions and to the content of the fantasies, understand their genesis and why they are occurring at that time, and, through this understanding, experience less distress and maladaptive behavior.

Psychodynamic Treatment Example In a PDP, the patient may have come to realize that he is especially vulnerable to having angry feelings about being controlled. He may have been sensitized to this issue by having strong angry feelings and thoughts of revenge when his therapist had to cancel an appointment on short notice. The patient responded by canceling his next appointment with the therapist on short notice and by having a fight with his wife that evening. When the therapist asked about the missed appointment, the patient was able to talk about his actions in the context of angry feelings he had toward the therapist and, in the past, toward his father. He was able to acknowledge his fantasy of being able to get revenge by canceling his appointment and understand how he displaced his anger toward his therapist onto his wife. He was also able to discuss how he had coped with these feelings in the past and developed increased insight into his vulnerabilities and maladaptive coping mechanisms.

Later in the month, when his boss asked him to change his vacation time, he recognized the same type of psychosocial stress and remembered that his angry reaction was probably more related to his father than to his boss's actual request. He was able to manage his initial angry reaction, his thought to "just say no," and told his boss he would think about it over the weekend.

When recommending psychotherapy, prescribe it like medication (Campbell, 2004). Be as specific as you can about the planned focus of psychotherapy, what psychological goals you have in mind, and which specific technique would be best suited for accomplishing these goals in this patient at this time. Analogous to pharmacotherapy, psychotherapy is available in a number of forms, each with its own indications and contraindications; it should be prescribed in a specific dose and frequency to address specific target symptoms; and, like any treatment, it may be associated with side effects. An example is shown in Table 7.3.

For beginning trainees, think about your patient and your psychological formulation. Think about psychological treatment interventions, including cognitive-behavioral and psychodynamic treatment interventions. For psychodynamically oriented treatments, consider discussing the types of transference thoughts or feelings you think the patient might develop toward the therapist and how discussion of those thoughts or feelings might help the patient.

For cognitive therapy, consider ways to help the patient manage strong emotions, identify automatic dysfunctional thoughts, negative core beliefs or cognitive distortions, and provide an example of a "homework" assignment that would help the patient begin to work on identifying and countering these beliefs.

For behavioral interventions, develop a simple intervention that might begin to reinforce adaptive behavior and extinguish maladaptive behavior.

Specify the duration (e.g., time-limited or open), format (e.g., individual, group, couples, or family therapy), and type (e.g., psychodynamic, cognitive, behavior, cognitive-behavioral

Table 7.3 Prescribing Psychotherapy Like Medication

THERAPY	TYPE OF INTERVENTION	SPECIFIC INTERVENTION	DOSE	FREQUENCY	TARGET SYMPTOMS	SIDE EFFECTS
Pharmacotherapy (medication)	Selective serotonin reuptake inhibitor (SSRI)	Fluoxetine	20 mg	Daily	Depressed mood, anhedonia, sleep disturbance	Nausea, diarrhea, sexual dysfunction
Psychotherapy	Individual	Psychodynamic	50 min	Weekly	Trauma, loss, low self-esteem	Anxiety, grief

[CBT], dialectical behavior [DBT], motivational enhancement [MET], interpersonal [IPT], supportive, psychoeducational, integrative) of psychotherapy to be employed.

As with the somatic treatments, it is prudent to have a brief description in mind for each of these modalities to share with patients, families, and health-care professionals.

SOCIAL TREATMENT PLAN

The social treatment plan is constructed in order to take maximum advantage of the patient's social strengths and to minimize the impact of psychosocial stressors on the patient's life. A cultural and spiritual assessment should be completed. Information from this assessment is then used to inform the treatment plan. For example, a psychosocial stressor in one culture or spiritual community may be perceived quite differently by those outside that culture or community.

Social Assessment

Based on the available data in the social formulation, determine whether specific assessments, such as functional or social assessments may be helpful.

Social Interventions

Review the categories in the social database once again in light of the information contained in the cultural and spiritual assessments. Consider which strengths should be mobilized and which specific interventions are needed to address each current stressor. Examples of social interventions for each of the 10 categories are shown in Table 7.4. Although some of the specific interventions will be psychological (e.g., psychotherapy), identification of a social stressor and referral for specific treatment (e.g., family therapy) is the appropriate social intervention.

Table 7.4   **Examples of Social Interventions**

Family
   Referral for psychotherapy for discussion of family difficulties
   Referral for family counseling
   Referral to the State Department of Child and Family Services

Friends/significant others
   Referral for psychotherapy for discussion of the loss or estrangement of friends
   Referral to a bereavement support group
   Social skills training to learn how to interact with others and to make friends

Social environment
   Referral to a community agency for recreational activities
   Referral to appropriate legal services for a discrimination lawsuit
   Referral to a senior volunteer agency

Education
   Referral to literacy volunteers to improve literacy
   Advocate for reinstatement at school following treatment for a mental disorder

Table 7.4 **Examples of Social Interventions** (*continued*)

Referral for psychological testing to determine whether a learning disorder is present

Work

Referral to the State Department of Labor for job retraining

Assistance in looking through want ads

Encourage continued work with job recruiters

Housing

Referral to Section 8 federal housing program

Assistance with accessing legal services to ensure constitutional rights are not being violated during an eviction

Discussion of privacy issues when living with a roommate

Income

Assistance in applying for job-related disability insurance

Referral to city and state welfare agencies

Assistance with strategizing about how best to approach family for money

Access to healthcare services

Referral to a social worker to assist in providing transportation

Ensure adequate primary care follow-up

Referral to a support group for a chronic medical condition

Legal problems/crime

Provide support during publicity about involvement in a high-profile lawsuit

Referral to a legal aid agency if indigent

Interact with lawyer (with patient's consent) to determine possible legal competency and, if necessary, appointment of a guardian or conservator of person or estate

Other

Intervene (with patient's consent) with other professional and nonprofessional caregiver(s) to help them provide better care to the patient

Referral for emergency assistance for disaster relief

Referral for counseling following exposure to a traumatic event

8

Prognosis

When clinicians are asked about a patient's prognosis, they frequently reply, "It's good" or "It's guarded." However, as you will see, prognosis is a much broader concept than this. Several factors must be considered in formulating a prognosis. These factors can be organized into two categories: disorder related and treatment related, as shown in Table 8.1.

Table 8.1   Prognostic Factors

Disorder-related factors

  Course

  Timing

  Social considerations

  Heredity

Treatment-related factors ("CRAPS")

  Compliance with treatment

  Response to prior treatment

  Availability of treatment

  Personality/defense mechanisms

  Social supports

The disorder-related factors are adapted from Morrison (1995). It is likely that beginning clinicians will need to consult a standard textbook of psychiatry to become familiar with the answers to these questions. This will again be time well spent, as questions about prognosis are important to patients and their families.

The first factor is *course*. Consider the following questions when addressing this factor: What is the usual longitudinal course of illness if the disorder is not treated? Is symptom reduction or remission expected? If remission is anticipated, what is the likelihood of recurrence? If not, is the disorder progressive?

The second factor is *timing*. Consider the following questions when addressing this factor: How rapid will the response be to the proposed treatments? How long will full recovery take? If the disorder is expected to recur, what will the anticipated interval be before the next episode?

The third factor is *social considerations*. Consider the following questions when addressing this factor: How is the illness expected to affect family life, job performance, and independence? Does the patient have adequate resources to access treatment? Will functioning return to a premorbid level? Will financial support be required? Will legal issues such as guardianship, civil commitment, or driving a car be affected?

The fourth factor is *heredity*. Consider the following question when addressing this factor: What was the course of illness like in other family members with the illness?

CRAPS, a mnemonic attributed to Robinson (Carlat, 1999), is useful for summarizing the treatment-related factors as depicted in Table 8.1.

9

Putting It All Together

In this chapter, a sample case study will be presented to illustrate the proper application of the Biopsychosocial Formulation Model.

IDENTIFYING INFORMATION

Mr. Doe is a 39-year-old married Caucasian man who lives with his wife and three daughters. He is a long-distance truck driver by trade.

REASON FOR REFERRAL

He was referred to the outpatient clinic by his primary care clinician for evaluation of "depression and anxiety."

CHIEF COMPLAINT

"I've been very stressed for a long time."

HISTORY OF PRESENT ILLNESS

Mr. Doe reports that his problems began 2 years ago when he had two myocardial infarctions followed by emergency coronary artery bypass grafting. He initially presented to an emergency department with chest pain, which the emergency physician attributed to anxiety. Mr. Doe was discharged home but presented again the next day with continuing chest pain and ruled in for a myocardial infarction. He was stabilized for several days in the hospital and then experienced recurrent chest pain. Cardiac isoenzymes were rising, so he was taken to the operating room for emergent coronary artery bypass grafting.

Mr. Doe says that his life has not been the same after this incident. He feels very angry that this happened to him at this early age, and he has become increasingly depressed and anxious about his declining health and function ("I'm falling apart, Doc"). His current symptoms, which worsened about 6 months ago, include a depressed and irritable mood, anhedonia, decreased appetite with 40-pound weight loss, poor sleep (2 to 3 hours of sleep per night), suicidal thoughts of driving off a bridge, decreased libido, and poor concentration. He has a persistent worry about dying suddenly. For example, he is afraid of falling asleep and not waking up in the morning. Mr. Doe reports thinking a lot about his father telling him he would be a failure and that has now turned out to be true. He can hear his father's voice saying this to him. He also reports that he has become very "snappy." He admits to frequent verbal altercations with his wife but denies any history of physical violence toward people or property. He denies any suicidal intent or homicidal ideation.

Mr. Doe related that he has also developed sudden, unexpected episodes of overwhelming anxiety accompanied by chest pain, shortness of breath, paresthesias of both arms, and feelings of doom since his myocardial infarctions. The symptoms usually remit in 20 minutes. He had two visits to the emergency department with no EKG changes and a stress thallium study that was negative. He was diagnosed with panic attacks, but continues to worry about this in light of his cardiac history. His primary care clinician started him on sertraline 2 months ago, but he has noticed no improvement in his depressive or anxiety symptoms.

PAST PSYCHIATRIC HISTORY/
SUBSTANCE ABUSE HISTORY

Mr. Doe denied any prior psychiatric history. He reported that he drank on a daily basis while in the service but denied any current alcohol or recreational drug use. He smoked a pack a day of cigarettes but reported that his use had doubled (2 PPD) in recent months because "It helps my nerves."

PAST MEDICAL HISTORY

Coronary artery disease, status post two myocardial infarctions and emergency coronary artery bypass grafting, hypertension, hypercholesterolemia, and a motor vehicle accident 6 months ago during which he struck his head on the steering wheel but did not sustain a loss of consciousness.

MEDICATIONS

Metoprolol 50 mg PO BID, amlodipine 5 mg PO QD, lovastatin 20 mg PO QD, sertraline 25 mg PO QD, ASA 325 mg PO QD, and NTG 0.4 mg SL PRN.

FAMILY HISTORY

Mr. Doe has two sisters and two brothers. One brother has hyperthyroidism. His father died of cancer at the age of 62, and his mother is alive and well at age 78. He denied any family history of mental disorders, with the exception of a cousin with alcohol dependence.

DEVELOPMENTAL AND SOCIAL HISTORY

Mr. Doe reports that his father was "very strict" and had "impossibly high standards." He recalls that his father constantly told him, "You'll never amount to anything." He denied any history of physical or sexual abuse, although he added that his father used frequent physical punishment (i.e., "whippings" with a belt) for minor transgressions. Mr. Doe joined the Marines while still in high school and later earned a GED while in the service. He served in the Marines for 4 years and was never in combat. He earned the rank of Sergeant and received an honorable discharge.

Mr. Doe is married and has three daughters, ages 2, 8, and 10. He reported being very proud of the large house and big truck he was able to purchase because he was so successful. The myocardial infarctions and cardiac surgery rendered him disabled for some time, which caused major financial problems that are still active. For example, he had to sell his home where he and his family were living at the time of his myocardial infarction and relocate to another state to live with his cousin. He stated that his cousin is an alcoholic and has caused Mr. Doe's family a great deal of distress by witnessing his binges. Mr. Doe has been trying to keep working, although he feels increasingly unsafe doing so because of his mental and physical conditions. His wife is studying to be a school bus driver so she can help support the family. He reported that his family "Couldn't be more supportive." He sees his mother, who lives alone in a large house, on a regular basis.

MENTAL STATUS EXAMINATION

Mr. Doe presented for the appointment well groomed and casually dressed. He was friendly and cooperative. His speech had a normal rate, volume, and prosody. His mood was described as "somewhat depressed" and "anxious." His affect was constricted but appropriate. He became tearful when talking about having to give up his work due to his physical and mental difficulties ("I've lost everything"). His thought process was logical and goal-directed. His thought content was remarkable for ruminations about his physical and mental states. He denied any obsessions, paranoid ideation, delusions, current suicidal or any homicidal ideation. He related that, at times, he hears his father's voice berating him but denied any visual hallucinations. His insight and judgment were good. He demonstrated an alert and nonfluctuating level of consciousness. He was fully oriented. He made one error in spelling "world" backward and two errors on serial sevens. He was able to register and recall three objects after 5 minutes of unrelated activity. His level of abstraction was good.

SCREENING LABORATORY DATA

Hemoglobin 14.7 g/dl, MCV 90.9 μm^3, WBC $9.1 \times 10^3/\mu l$, platelet count $307 \times 10^3/\mu l$, Na^+ 139 mmol/L, K^+ 4.2 mmol/L, creatinine 1.3 mg/dl, liver function tests WNL, HDL 35 mg/dl, LDL 142 mg/dl, TSH 0.9 $\mu U/ml$.

NARRATIVE SUMMARY

In summary, this is a 39-year-old married Caucasian man who is referred for psychiatric evaluation by his primary care clinician for depression and anxiety. His chief complaint is "I've been very stressed for a long time." The patient is a long-distance truck driver, currently living with his wife and three daughters at his cousin's home.

He reports that his problems began 2 years ago when he presented to an emergency department with chest pain. The emergency physician thought this was due to anxiety and discharged the patient home. He returned the following day with continuing chest pain and was diagnosed with a myocardial infarction. The patient had a stable hospital course for several days but then experienced recurrent chest pain associated with rising cardiac isoenzymes. He was taken to the operating room where he underwent coronary artery bypass grafting.

The patient reports that his life has not been the same following this incident. He feels angry that this had to happen to him at this early age, and he has become increasingly depressed and anxious about his declining health and function. The patient also reported that his symptoms worsened about 6 months ago. He currently endorses:

- Mood symptoms, including an irritable (he reported that he has become very "snappy") and depressed mood, anhedonia, insomnia with 2 to 3 hours of sleep a night, anorexia with a 40-pound weight loss, difficulty with concentration, feelings of guilt and worthlessness (he reported that he has been thinking a lot about his father telling him he would be a failure and that now that has turned out to be true), decreased libido, and intermittent suicidal ideation in which he considers "giving up" or "driving off a bridge." The patient specifically denied any current active suicidal ideation or any homicidal ideation.

- Anxiety symptoms, including an anxious mood, persistent worry about dying suddenly (he reported that he is afraid of falling asleep and not waking up in the morning), and panic attacks consisting of sudden episodes of severe anxiety accompanied by chest pain, shortness of breath, paresthesias of both arms, and "feeling as though life is ending." The panic attacks are not situationally bound or predisposed and remit within 20 minutes. Medical evaluation, including a negative stress thallium study, has revealed no cardiac basis for the symptoms. However, he continues to worry about this. His father's admonitions have become ruminations and should also be considered a symptom of anxiety. The patient denied any clear PTSD symptoms.

- Psychotic symptoms, including hearing his father's voice telling him that he would be a failure. There were no delusions evident during this evaluation. However, keep in mind that his father's admonitions have the potential of reaching a delusional level over time.

- Cognitive symptoms, including difficulty with concentration.

- Substance-related symptoms, including use of nicotine. He reported a doubling of his use of cigarettes, but specifically denied any current use of alcohol or recreational drugs.

PREDISPOSING, OR CONTRIBUTING, BIOLOGICAL, PSYCHOLOGICAL, AND SOCIAL FACTORS

Predisposing, or contributing, factors will be reviewed from biological, psychological, and social perspectives. With regard to biological contributors to this patient's clinical presentation, he denied any family history of mental disorders, including substance abuse, with the exception of his cousin, who has a history of alcohol abuse. Accordingly, his current symptoms are unlikely to be the result of a genetic diathesis.

However, the patient has several physical illnesses that are associated with mental disorders, including hypercholesterolemia, hypertension, and coronary artery disease with two myocardial infarctions and coronary artery bypass grafting. Cerebrovascular disease is a common comorbid condition with coronary artery disease and may be a biological contributor to the current clinical presentation. Neuropsychological deficits have been documented following coronary artery bypass grafting, and this is a possible explanation for the mild cognitive deficits apparent on the mental status examination. It would be prudent to complete the cognitive portion of the mental status examination, including assessment of language, visuospatial construction, and abstraction, in order to identify other potential deficits. The patient also related a history of head trauma without loss of consciousness. However, loss of consciousness is neither a sufficient nor necessary condition for traumatic brain injury. Accordingly, this may be a contributor as well. The patient's current medications include three classes of drugs associated with mood symptoms, including a lipophilic beta-blocker (metoprolol), a calcium channel antagonist (amlodipine), and an HMG-CoA reductase inhibitor (lovastatin). The onset or exacerbation of symptoms should be reviewed with respect to the initiation or increases in the dosage of these medications.

From a psychological perspective, the patient experienced a significant disruption in his psychological development as a result of having a very strict father with impossibly high standards. The father's admonition that the patient would never amount to anything has become a distressing rumination in the patient's current clinical presentation. Although the patient denied any history of physical or sexual abuse, he stated that his father would administer punishment by whipping him with a belt. This suggests that the father engaged in other behaviors consistent with the traditional image of men being tough. It is interesting that the patient joined the Marines while still in high school and later became a truck driver. Both of these career choices are consistent with wanting to be perceived as tough. It is likely that the patient sees himself as deficient or defective in some way and has compensated for this by adopting a strong work ethic and priding himself on being the main provider for his family. He is now experiencing considerable shame, guilt, and anger, the latter being displaced onto his wife, whom with he admits having frequent verbal altercations (one wonders whether he is using repression or denial when he states that his family couldn't be more supportive). It is also likely that he finds authority figures untrustworthy, given his father's behavior as well as the emergency physician's misdiagnosis of the patient's chest pain. Recurrent themes are likely to revolve around issues of trust, but also around issues of initiative. The patient's behavior is consistent with difficulties with the phallic-oedipal phase of psychosexual development. Phallic narcissism is manifested by the need to engage in masculine activities and be perceived as a "real man" in an effort to regulate self-esteem. The patient's avoidance of applying for disability benefits and decision to relocate to his cousin's home instead of his mother's are behaviors that are consistent with this hypothesis. It is also likely that he will minimize his symptoms on this basis. From a cognitive perspective, the patient manifests a number of cognitive distortions and errors in logic, including all-or-nothing thinking and overgeneralization, believing that he is a complete failure. Behavioral considerations include an aversive conditioned response to anything that might be perceived as unmanly. These responses may be viewed as paired associations based on prior experience with an overbearing father. An example would be the avoidance of any form of support from his mother because "real men" don't rely on their mothers. Regular exercise has been shown to enhance mood and would be a positively reinforcing intervention.

The patient is facing several social challenges at the present time, including marital discord, limited social supports, living in an alcoholic cousin's home, employment difficulties, physical disability, and financial hardship. His social strengths include a basic education (GED), no current legal problems, and access to health care. From a cultural perspective, the patient is a blue-collar worker. Although he may be overtly compliant with recommendations from authority figures, he may believe that these individuals do not understand his needs because they are not like him, leading to a failure to comply. The assignment of a female clinician or perhaps someone from a foreign country or minority group to his care would likely exacerbate the problem. Consistent with his psychological makeup, he is likely to be stoic and minimize his symptoms.

MULTIAXIAL DIFFERENTIAL DIAGNOSIS

With regard to differential diagnosis, diagnoses that should be considered on Axis I include the following:

- Major Depressive Disorder, Single Episode, Severe, With Psychotic Features
- Bipolar I Disorder, Severe, With Psychotic Features, Most Recent Episode Mixed
- Panic Disorder With and Without Agoraphobia

- Mood/Psychotic Disorder Due to a General Medical Condition
- Nicotine Dependence
- We would also note a past history of Alcohol Abuse (*remember not to "orphan" any data*) and keep alcohol-induced mood/psychotic disorder in the differential pending corraboration of the patient's history

Although his symptoms are in response to a severe stressor, we would not consider the diagnosis of Adjustment Disorder With Mixed Anxiety and Depressed Mood, as his symptoms are too severe, or Posttraumatic Stress Disorder, as he specifically denied any symptoms referable to this (*remember to consider pertinent negatives*). Given the available information at this time, our presumptive diagnosis would be Major Depressive Disorder With Psychotic Features.

We would defer any diagnosis on Axis II on the basis of this single evaluation. However, we would make a mental note of the "snappy" behavior he describes, as this may be a maladaptive form of coping for him that predated the depression.

On Axis III, we would list hypercholesterolemia, hypertension, coronary artery disease status post two myocardial infarctions and emergent coronary artery bypass grafting in

March of 1998, and a motor vehicle accident with head injury, but no loss of consciousness, 6 months ago.

We would list marital discord, limited social supports, living in an alcoholic cousin's home, employment difficulties, physical disability, and financial hardship on Axis IV.

On Axis V, we would give the patient a current GAF score of 42, given the severity of his symptoms. Based on the available information, the highest GAF in the past year is unlikely to have been higher than 55.

RISK ASSESSMENT

The patient has a number of dynamic risk factors for suicide, including depressed mood, potential loss of rational thought with the deprecating ruminations and auditory hallucinations, limited social supports, and, arguably, physical disability. Although he experienced suicidal ideation and intermittently thought about driving off a bridge, he has no prior history of suicidal behavior and denied any current suicidal ideation. Accordingly, his suicide risk is moderate, and he should be closely followed on an outpatient basis (i.e., seen at least once a week until his symptoms begin to show clear improvement). With regard to violence risk, the patient has no prior history of violence and denied any thoughts of harming others. Accordingly, his violence risk is judged to be low.

BIOPSYCHOSOCIAL TREATMENT PLAN

The biological assessment ("reversible workup") should consist of a routine physical examination, including a complete neurological examination, and laboratory studies to rule out reversible causes for this patient's clinical presentation. These would include a complete blood count with differential; blood sugar; electrolytes; BUN; creatinine; calcium; liver function tests including albumin, AST, ALT, alkaline phosphatase, and bilirubin; TSH; vitamin B_{12}; folate; RPR; and urine toxicology screen. If there were any risks factors associated with HIV (for example, unprotected sex with prostitutes) or exposure to ticks (Lyme disease is endemic in certain areas in the United States), HIV and Lyme antibody screens should be ordered as well. Given the patient's past history of extracorporeal circulation during coronary artery bypass grafting, if the cognitive deficits persisted, it would be prudent to order a brain MRI with gadolinium even in the presence of a normal neurological examination. There is no indication for outside consultation at this time.

With regard to biological interventions, the antihypertensive regimen should be reviewed with the patient's primary care clinician to ascertain whether any reductions in dosage or changes to drugs not associated with mood symptoms (for example, a hydrophilic beta-blocker such as atenolol) can be made. The current dose of sertraline is unlikely to have any effect on his symptoms. It should be gradually increased, as tolerated, while the target symptoms are monitored. Given his history of panic attacks, the dose can be increased in 25 mg increments to a total of at least 100 mg. Further adjustments can then be made on the basis of target symptoms. The results of the laboratory studies and neuroimaging should be carefully reviewed and any abnormalities promptly addressed.

From a psychological perspective, no testing is indicated based on the current information. However, neuropsychological testing would be ordered in the event that informal mental status testing turned up further cognitive deficits, or if the current deficits persisted once the other symptoms remitted. A functional assessment and vocational aptitude testing would be useful studies given the patient's current disability.

Weekly individual cognitive-behavioral psychotherapy should begin at the earliest convenience, as this, in combination with pharmacotherapy, has been shown to result in the highest rate of symptoms remission. The therapy should focus on the patient's current cognitive distortions. Marital therapy may be a useful intervention once the patient is more stable.

From a social perspective, involvement of supportive family members in the patient's care can be exceedingly helpful. Results of the functional assessment and aptitude tests should be reviewed with the patient, and a collaborative effort may then be undertaken to address his current employment difficulties. This may involve additional education in a community college or technical school, or enrollment in a formal vocational rehabilitation program. The current housing arrangement should be reviewed with the patient and his family, as this appears to be an additional stressor. Alternatives include relocating to his mother's spacious home or exploring the availability of subsidized (Section 8) housing through the Veteran's Administration. Finally, assistance should be provided with completing the requisite applications for general assistance and disability payments, as these will ease the financial hardship.

PROGNOSIS

The overall prognosis for this patient is fair to good. It is likely that his physical disability will continue to be a problem in the short to intermediate term. However, his symptoms should respond favorably to the combination of pharmacotherapy and psychotherapy. Gradual improvement of the social stressors will also have a salutary effect on his clinical presentation.

APPENDIX A

Other Psychodynamic Perspectives[*]

Three other psychodynamic perspectives are worthy of consideration. Remember, the more tools you have in your toolbox,

---

[*] Adapted from Gabbard, 2005. The first component is ego *strengths and weaknesses*. A thorough assessment of the major ego functions includes specific consideration of each of the following: relation to reality, thought processes, control and regulation of instinctual drives, judgment, defense mechanisms, object (interpersonal) relations, autonomous ego functions, synthetic ego functions, and psychological mindedness. Descriptions of the major ego functions are provided in Appendix B.

the better prepared you will be to analyze a problem, in this case, your patient's maladaptive pattern of thinking, feeling, and behaving. The three other psychodynamic perspectives include ego psychology, object relations, and self-psychology.

The first perspective is based on Anna Freud's ego psychology (Gabbard, 2005; Pine, 1990; Sadock and Sadock, 1994). This theory focuses on characteristics of the ego depicted in Table A.1.

The first component is ego strengths and weaknesses. An evaluation of ego functions can contribute to a decision regarding whether a patient requires treatment in an inpatient setting.

The second component is *defense mechanisms and conflicts.* Although analysts disagree on the total number of defense mechanisms, most agree with Freud's assessment that defense mechanisms must possess the following properties: (a) they manage instinct, drive, and mood; (b) they are unconscious; (c) they are discrete; (d) they are dynamic and reversible; and (e) they can be adaptive or pathological. Defense mechanisms may be categorized into primary (primitive) and secondary (higher-order) defensive processes. Their descriptions are provided in chapter 3.

The third component is *relationship to the superego.* When assessing this aspect of psychological functioning, pose the

Table A.1 Characteristics of the Ego

Strengths and weaknesses
Defense mechanisms and conflicts
Relationship to the superego

following question: "Is the superego a rigid and punitive over-seer of the ego or is there a flexible and harmonious interaction between them?"

The second perspective is based on Klein, Fairbairn, Winnicott and others' object relations theory (Gabbard, 2005; Pine, 1990; Sadock and Sadock, 2004; St. Clair, 1999). This theory focuses on the quality of object* relations as depicted in Table A.2.

The first component is *interpersonal relationships*. Consideration should be given to all meaningful interactions with others, including childhood relationships, the real and transferential relationship with the therapist, and current relationships.

The second component is *level of integration (maturity) of internal object relations*. When assessing this aspect of psychological functioning, pose the following question: "Are others seen as need-gratifying part objects or as whole objects with their own needs and concerns? Are they viewed ambivalently

---

* The use of the term "object" is unfortunate because it leads to considerable confusion. In most instances, and for the current application, object refers to person. Therefore, object relations can be interpreted as interpersonal relations.

Table A.2   Quality of Object Relations

Interpersonal relationships
Level of integration (maturity) of internal object relations
Object constancy

with both good and bad qualities or as idealized ('all good') or devalued ('all bad')?"

The third component is *object constancy*. When assessing this aspect of psychological functioning, ask, "Can the patient tolerate being apart from significant others by summoning up a soothing internal image of the person?" If the answer is affirmative, they attained object constancy; if it is negative, they have not.

The third perspective is based on Kohut's theory of self-psychology (Gabbard 2005; Pine 1990; Sadock and Sadock 2004; St. Clair 1999). This theory focuses on characteristics of the self, as depicted in Table A.3.

The first component is *self-esteem and self-cohesiveness*. This refers to the durability and cohesiveness of the self. When assessing this aspect of psychological functioning, pose the following questions: "Is the self prone to fragmentation

Table A.3   Characteristics of the Self

Self-esteem and self-cohesiveness
Self-continuity
Self-boundaries

in response to minor slights? Does the patient need to be in the spotlight continually to receive affirming (i.e., 'mirroring') responses or bask in the presence of an idealized other (i.e., 'idealizing' response)? Are the patient's self-object needs satisfied in a mature manner (i.e., in the context of a mutually satisfying long-term relationship)?" The second component is *self-continuity*. When assessing this aspect of psychological functioning, ask, "Is the patient much the same over time, regardless of external circumstances, or is there generalized identity diffusion?" The third component is *self-boundaries*. Assessment of this aspect of psychological functioning is made by asking, "Can the patient clearly separate his or her own mental contents from those of others or is there a general blurring of self-object boundaries? Are the patient's body boundaries intact or do they have to engage in self-mutilation to define the skin boundary?"

APPENDIX B

*Major Ego Functions**

RELATION TO REALITY

The mediation between the internal world and external reality is a crucial function of the ego. The relationship with the

---

*   Adapted from Gabbard, 2005; McWilliams, 1994; Pine, 1990; Sadock and Sadock, 2004.

outside world can be divided into three aspects: sense of reality, reality testing, and adaptation to reality. The sense of reality develops in concert with the infant's dawning awareness of bodily sensations. The ability to distinguish what is outside the body from what is inside is an essential aspect of the sense of reality, and disturbances of body boundaries, such as depersonalization, reflect impairment in that ego function.

Reality testing is an ego function of paramount importance in that it differentiates psychotic persons from non-psychotic persons. Reality testing refers to the capacity to distinguish internal fantasy from external reality. That function of ego gradually develops in parallel with the increasing dominion of the reality principal over the pleasure principle.

The third aspect, adaptation to reality, involves the ability to use one's resources to develop effective responses to changing circumstances on the basis of previous experiences with reality. One may perceive reality accurately but not use one's full resources to make an informed judgment about the necessary response. In that sense, adaptation is closely linked to the concept of mastery with respect to control of drives and accomplishment of external tasks. Adaptation to reality is also intimately connected with defensive functions of the ego. One commonly calls on a variety of defensive maneuvers to master situations that may produce anxiety or other affects.

For example, to deal with overwhelming trauma, one may use temporary denial to get through the crisis.

THOUGHT PROCESSES

The adequacy of the processes that actively guide and sustain thought, including attention, concentration, anticipation, concept formation, memory, and language is considered in this ego function. Thought processes can be primary or secondary. Primary process thinking is unconscious, preverbal, prerational, and egocentric. Examples of primary thought processes include dreams and psychosis. Secondary process thinking is conscious, verbal, rational, and goal directed. Adults normally display secondary (logical) thought processes. The extent of relative primary–secondary process influences on thought should always be assessed.

CONTROL AND REGULATION OF INSTINCTUAL DRIVES

The development of the capacity to delay or postpone drive discharge, like the capacity to test reality, is closely related to the progression in early childhood from the pleasure principle to the reality principle. That capacity is also an essential aspect of the ego's role as mediator between the id and the outside world. Part of the infant's socialization to the external world is the acquisition of language and secondary process or logical thinking, both of which assist in the control of instinctual drives. The capacity to think in a logical and abstract manner allows for the representation of drives in fantasy, which may circumvent the need to discharge them in action.

The ego's capacity to regulate thinking and to control drive discharge is intimately connected with its defensive functioning. One example of the linkage between control of drives and defensive functioning can be seen in the ego's use of signal affects. Affect states such as guilt, anxiety, shame, and depression serve as signals of the potential breakthrough of threatening impulses from the unconscious. Those signals then act to mobilize defenses in the ego to prevent the breakthrough. That function of the ego is also instrumental in building a capacity to tolerate pain, anxiety, and frustration within manageable limits.

JUDGMENT

A closely related ego function is judgment, which involves the ability to anticipate the consequences of one's actions. As with the control and regulation of instinctual drives, judgment develops in parallel with the growth of secondary process thinking. The ability to think logically allows for an assessment of how one's contemplated behavior may affect others. The consequences to oneself can also be ascertained through the use of secondary process thinking. The ego function of judgment may assist regulatory aspects of the ego in the avoidance of impulse discharge.

DEFENSE MECHANISMS

Defense mechanisms are habitual patterns of dealing with stress (see chapter 3).

OBJECT (INTERPERSONAL) RELATIONS

The significance of object relationships in normal psychological development and in psychiatric disorders was not fully appreciated until relatively late in the evolution of classical psychoanalysis. The capacity to form mutually satisfying relationships is, in part, related to patterns of internalization stemming from early interactions with parents and other significant figures. That ability is also a fundamental function of the ego in that satisfying relatedness depends on the ability to integrate positive and negative aspects of others and oneself and to maintain an internal sense of others, even in their absence.

AUTONOMOUS EGO FUNCTIONS

A direct outgrowth of the work of Hartmann, the primary autonomous functions refer to rudimentary apparatuses that are present at birth and that develop independently of intrapsychic conflict between drives and defenses, provided that what Hartmann referred to as an *average expectable environment* is available to the infant. The functions include perception, learning, intelligence, intuition, language, thinking, comprehension, and motility. In the course of development, some of those conflict-free aspects of the ego may eventually become involved in conflict if they encounter opposing forces.

SYNTHETIC EGO FUNCTIONS

First described by Herman Nunberg in 1931, the synthetic function refers to the ego's capacity to integrate diverse elements into an overall unity. Different aspects of oneself and others, for example, are synthesized into a consistent representation that endures over time. The function also involves organizing, coordinating, and generalizing or simplifying large amounts of data.

PSYCHOLOGICAL MINDEDNESS

This ego function refers to the ability of the individual to both monitor and evaluate thoughts, emotions, and behavior.

Appendix C

*A Glossary of Psychoanalytic Terms**

Autism   Normal autism refers to the first month of life when an infant is psychologically undifferentiated and is turned inward.

Bad object   An object that frustrates and also receives a projection of destructive instincts from the individual in relation to it.

---

*   Adapted from Gabbard, 2005; McWilliams, 1994; Pine, 1990; Sadock and Sadock, 2004; St. Clair, 1999.

Cathexis   An investment of instinctual or emotional energy.

Cohesive self and fragmented self   The feeling of wholeness versus that of being in parts or the feeling of a loss of continuity.

Death instinct   A drive toward destruction that can be turned inward toward the self or toward the outside world in an aggressive way.

Defense mechanism   A process by which the ego protects itself from threatening thoughts and feelings.

Depressed position   A Kleinian term for a developmental stage that peaks at about the sixth month during which the infant fears destruction and the loss of the loved object.

Development   Growth as a sequence of stages, either from an instinctual perspective or from the perspective of relationships with persons in the environment.

Drive   Instinctual force (sexual and aggressive) that moves a person to action.

Drive derivatives   A transformation or distortion of a drive so that the drive takes a new form, such as that which might be manifested in a dream symbol.

Ego   From a conceptual rather than experiential viewpoint, that part of the personality that has consciousness and performs various functions, such as keeping in contact with reality.

Ego boundary   That which gives a sense of (a) the distinction between oneself and external objects, or (b) the distinction between the mind's conscious thoughts and feelings and repressed thoughts and feelings.

Ego dystonic   Feelings, ideas, and actions that are not in harmony with an individual's values and principles and, consequently, cause anxiety.

Ego functions   Operations assigned to the ego, such as maintaining contact with reality, perception, regulating drives, executing the wishes of the id, defending against impulses, relating to objects, and so forth.

Ego ideal   An aspect of the superego that has an image of perfection that the individual holds up for him- or herself.

Ego syntonic   Feelings, ideas, and actions that are compatible and in harmony with one's values and principles.

Energy   The forces that motivate or move a person toward activity.

Externalize   To mentally or imaginatively locate one's wish or feeling as being outside oneself, such as a child being afraid of monsters in the dark.

Facilitating environment   Persons who provide what an infant needs, especially a sense of narcissistic omnipotence necessary for development.

Fixation   A stage of development in which getting gratification or relating to people is highly energized either by excessive satisfaction or excessive frustration; the result is that the individual persists in this pattern of getting gratification or relating to people.

Genital stage   The last phase of instinctual development, with the implication that the chosen love object is another person and that the individual has a biological capacity for intercourse and orgasm.

Good-enough mother   One who sufficiently meets the needs of her child, especially by responding to the spontaneous gesture of the child in a way that fosters healthy narcissism.

Good object   An object that gratifies and also receives the projection of libidinal instinct from the individual in relation to it.

Holding environment   A safe, nurturing environment (or person), with an infant protected from excessive internal and external demands and stimulation.

Hysteria   Suggests, among other qualities, that a person is excitable, emotional, and talkative, but poorly observant of inner feelings.

Id   From a conceptual point of view, a structure of the mind that is associated with instinctual drives and seeks to reduce tension by gratifying those drives.

Identification   A process by which an individual becomes like or gets an identity from another.

Identity   A sense of being the same unique self over time.

Incorporation   A form of introjection suggesting a taking into the mind through the bodily process of swallowing.

Instinct   A drive or biological urge to take action.

Internal object   A phantasy or image of an object.

Internalization   A process by which an individual transforms characteristics of the environment into inner characteristics.

Introjection   An assimilation of an object or its demands into the ego, or the assimilation of the object representation into the self-representation.

Latency   A period in development, extending approximately from 7 years of age to puberty, when psychosocial forces or libidinal interests are active.

Libido   A term for sexual drive energy, not sexual desire.

Masochism   Gaining sexual satisfaction by suffering pain.

Model   A set of concepts explaining a complex reality.

Narcissism   An investment or concentration of energy or interest in the self. In traditional psychoanalysis, narcissism refers to a withdrawal of libido from external objects and an investment in the self. Healthy narcissism for self-psychology implies the development of self-esteem through a relationship with a self object.

Neurosis   A disorder affecting only part of the personality, implying relatively stable and undifferentiated psychic structures, and with the conflict primarily between the ego and the impulses of the id.

Object   The "other" involved in a relationship or, from an instinctual point of view, that from which the instinct gets gratification.

Object choice   Selection of a person as a loved object.

Object relatedness   Interpersonal relationships as they exist externally.

Object relations   Interpersonal relationships as they are represented intrapsychically.

Object representation   An intrapsychic image of the other in relation to the self.

Obsessive   A way of thinking that is repetitive, insistent, and inhibiting of thought and action.

Oedipus complex   A developmental situation during which the child moves from a dyadic relation with the mother to a triadic relationship with both parents; the child identifies with the parent of the same sex and chooses the parent of the opposite sex as a loved object.

Oral stage   In Freud's model, the first stage of development, which is characterized by libidinal interests centering in the mouth.

Paranoid-schizoid position   A developmental position postulated by Klein that peaks about the third month of life and is characterized by aggression and feelings of persecution.

Part object   When only one aspect of an object is perceived, such as goodness or badness, gratifying or frustrating.

Phallic stage   The third stage of development in Freud's model, approximately from ages 3 to 5, characterized by increasing interest in the genitals.

Phantasy   The mental imagery expressing instinctual drives; different from whimsical fantasies or daydreams.

Pleasure principle   A regulatory norm for activity that usually involves an uninhibited effort to reduce drive tension and gratify needs; occurs earlier than the reality principle.

Practicing subphase   A period during the separation–individuation phase of development, roughly beginning from 10 to 12 months and lasting through 16 to 18 months, when the child experiences exuberance in being able to distance him- or herself from mother by walking.

Pregenital   The early stages of development when gratification is primarily oriented in the child's own body and to the mother only insofar as she provides gratification.

Preoedipal   The characteristics and interests of the early stages of development before the oedipal complex.

Primary process   A mode of thinking characterized by wishful phantasy and association as found in dreams.

Projection   To imaginatively put onto another what belongs to oneself so that one's subjective reality becomes objectified and externalized.

Projective identification   Imaginatively splitting off part of oneself and attributing that part to another for the sake of controlling the other.

Psyche   The mind or mental life.

Psychic mechanism   A process of the mind with a specific function, such as protecting consciousness from inner dangers.

Psychosis   A serious disturbance characterized by a collapse of psychic structures and a distortion in the perception of reality.

Rapprochement   A subphase of the separation–individuation phase of development; roughly the period from 18 to 24 months of age, during which time the child experiences an increase in helplessness and a resurgence of the need for closeness to the mother.

Reality principle   A regulatory norm that modifies the pleasure principle and aims to keep the activity of the ego in line with the demands of social reality rather than with instinctual demands.

Representation   An affective mental structure made up of a multitude of impressions and feelings; a psychological structure that differs from a merely visual or perceptual mental image.

Repression   The defense by which unwanted thoughts and feelings are kept out of awareness.

Schizoid   Characterized by having intense needs for objects but with fear of closeness with the same objects;

the schizoid personality feels isolated, meaningless, and withdrawn.

Secondary process   Mental activity proper to the ego — that is, logical, orderly, and in touch with reality.

Self   A complex term with several frames of reference; can refer to person as subject as distinguished from objects in the environment, the person who I am for myself, or the representation or image of the self-contained in the ego.

Selfobject   Kohut's term for the person used in the service of the self or experienced as part of the self, especially with regard to fostering esteem and a sense of well-being.

Separation–individuation   A phase of development and a process in which the child increasingly disengages from psychological fusion with the mother and increasingly gains a sense of being an autonomous person.

Splitting   A developmental and defensive process of keeping incompatible feelings apart and separate.

Structure   Stable, inner psychological patterns.

Superego   Inner controls or ideals that become established at about 6 or 7 years of age.

Symbiotic phase   Margaret Mahler's term for the developmental period from approximately the second to sixth months of life, during which time the infant phantasizes that the infant and his or her mother are fused in a dual entity with a common boundary.

Transference   Assigning feelings from a past relationship to a present relationship with a therapist.

Transitional object   Something that a child uses for comfort and security as the child moves from one level of emotional development to another; a teddy bear, for example.

Transmuting internalization   Kohut's term for the process by which functions of persons in the environment are internalized by a child as inner structures and functions.

True self and false self   Winnicott's terms for the feeling of being real, whole, and spontaneous as opposed to the sense of compliancy and the covering of one's real needs.

Unconscious   Thoughts and feelings out of awareness of the conscious ego.

Whole object   Perception of an object as a whole person, as a love object, with the implication that the perceiver has the developmental capacity for ambivalence and is thus capable of accepting both good and bad qualities in the object.

APPENDIX D

The Biopsychosocial Formulation
Manual Database Record

ID: FH:
RFR/CC:

HPI:
Symptoms:

Precipitants:
                              DH/SH:

PPH:
                              Functional Assessment

SAH:
                              MSE:

PMH:

                              PE/Neuro:
Meds:

                              Diagnostic Studies:

Allergies:

SYMPTOM FILTER:

Mood	Anxiety	Psychosis	Somatic	Cognitive	Substance	Personality	Other

FORMULATION:

Biological	Psychological	Social
Genetics, physical conditions, medication, substances	Psychodynamic, cognitive or behavioral	Current stressors Social strengths Cultural assess-ment

DIFFERENTIAL DIAGNOSIS:
Axis I

Axis II
Axis III
Axis IV
Axis V GAF=

Risk assessment:

BIOPSYCHOSOCIAL TREATMENT PLAN

Biological	Psychological	Social

Prognosis:

References

1. American Psychiatric Association. (2000). *Diagnostic and statistical manual of mental disorders* (4th ed., text revision; *DSM-IV-TR*). Washington, DC: Author.

2. Beck, J. B. (1985). *Cognitive therapy: Basics and beyond.* New York: Guilford Press.

3. Campbell, W. H. (2004). Revised 'SAD PERSONS' helps assess suicide risk. *Current Psychiatry, 3,* 102.

4. Campbell, W. H. (2004). 'Prescribing' psychotherapy as if it were medication. *Current Psychiatry, 3,* 66-71.

5. Carlat, D. J. (1999). *The psychiatric interview: A practical guide.* Philadelphia: Lippincott, Williams & Wilkins.

6. Engel, G. L. (1977). The need for a new medical model: a challenge for biomedicine. *Science, 196,* 129–136.

7. Engel, G. L. (1980). The clinical application of the biopsychosocial model. *American Journal of Psychiatry, 137,* 535–544.

8. Gabbard, G. O. (2005). *Psychodynamic psychiatry in clinical practice* (4th ed.). Washington, DC: American Psychiatric Press.

9. McWilliams, N. (1994). *Psychoanalytic diagnosis. Understanding personality structure in the clinical process.* New York: Guilford Press.

10. Morrison, J. (1995). *The first interview: Revised for DSM-IV.* New York: Guilford Press.

11. Patterson, W. M., Dohn, H. H., Bird, J., & Patterson, G. (1983). Evaluation of suicidal patients: The SAD PERSONS scale. *Psychosomatics, 24,* 343–349.

12. Pine, F. (1990). *Drive, ego, object, & self. A synthesis for clinical work.* New York: Basic Books.

13. Sadock, B. J., & Sadock, V. A. (Eds.). (2004). *Kaplan & Sadock's comprehensive textbook of psychiatry* (8th ed.). Philadelphia: Lippincott Williams & Wilkins.

14. St. Clair, M. (1999). *Object relations and self psychology: An introduction* (3rd ed.). Pacific Grove, CA: Brooks/Cole.

Index

terminology, 145–153
themes, identification of, 25–30
vulnerabilities, 93–94
Psychological themes, 25–30
Psychotherapy, *see also* CBT; PDP
cognitive behavioral (CBT), 97–98
psychodynamic (PDP), 98–100
Punishment, 60

R

Rationalization, 50
Reaction formation, 50
Reality, relation to, 137–139
Reasoning, emotional, 57
Regression, 51
Reinforcement, 59–60
Relationships
difficulties, recurrent, 28–29
interpersonal, 133
object (interpersonal), 141–142
Repetition compulsion, 39
Repression, 51
Revelatory statements and behavior,
29–30
Risk assessment, 75–84
case study, 126–127
formulation, 81–83
risk reduction plan, 83–84
suicide, 76–78
violence, 78–79

S

SAD PERSONS/PERSONAS, 76–
78; *see also* Suicide
Self-psychology, 134–135
SIG: E-CAPS, 16; *see also* Depression
Skinner, B.F., 59
Social formulation, 63–70
database, 63–66
social environment, 65
social history, 23–24

Somatic treatment, *see* Treatments
Somatization, 52; *see also* Medical
history
Spiritual assessment, 66–70
Splitting, 46
Statements
imperative, 59
revelatory, 29–30
Stress, dealing with, 33–36
Stressors (psychosocial), 31–33, 94–96
Sublimation, 52
Substance abuse, 14
Suicide, 76–78
Superego, 132; *see also* Ego
Suppression, 52
Symptom Filter, 10, 15–16, 71–72
Synthetic functions, *see* Ego

T

Terminology, 145–153
Themes
developmental, 38–39
identification of, 25–30
Treatments
biological, 86–91
biopsychosocial, 85–105
case study, 127–129
psychological, 91–103
social, 103–105
somatic, 88–91
Tunnel vision, 59

V

Violence
affective ("hot"), 82–83
predatory ("cold"), 83
risk assessment, 78–79

W

Work, 65
Workup, reversible, 86–88

CD Contents

Printed in the United States
by Baker & Taylor Publisher Services